DEPARTMENT OF HEALTH AND SOCIAL SECURITY

Report of the Review
of
Rampton Hospital

Presented to Parliament by the Secretary of State for Social Services
by Command of Her Majesty
[November 1980]

LONDON
HER MAJESTY'S STATIONERY OFFICE
£6.70 net

Cmnd 8073

ISBN 0 10 180730 9

REPORT OF THE RAMPTON HOSPITAL MANAGEMENT REVIEW TEAM

To The Right Honourable Patrick Jenkin MP
Secretary of State for Social Services.

6 October 1980

Dear Secretary of State

Rampton Hospital

I am pleased to send you the Report of the Rampton Hospital Review Team. The fact that I am able to do this within the timetable you set is due to the unremitting hard work of the Team members and their secretary Mr Robin Orton assisted in the last months by Mr Owen Thorpe.

Members of the Team with nursing medical or hospital experience have spent many weeks living at the hospital. We have a full and thorough knowledge of Rampton's working and are in a unique position to assess what is good and what is bad there. We have found much that is worthy of praise and have set this out in our Report. We have a real appreciation of the tireless care and attention which the staff at Rampton give to a class of patient for whom much of society asks little more than that the patients be kept safely locked-up.

Yet there is no doubt that changes need to be made at Rampton. The hospital appears to have been in a backwater and the main currents of thought about the care of mental patients have passed it by.

We have discussed our principal findings with management and staff. It is encouraging that they appear to accept the need to re-examine traditional Rampton attitudes, practices and régimes. There are signs that the institutional inertia of the hospital is being overcome.

Nevertheless we are convinced that the momentum of change will only gather speed if Rampton can have a much longer period of attention than we can give to it. That is why we wish to hand over our work to a Review Board which we recommend that you should set up. Assisted by the appointment of a new Medical Director, the Review Board should be able to make Rampton a better place for both patients and staff in a way which we are not constituted to achieve.

Our report lays the foundation, but others must build upon it, not least the ordinary member of staff at Rampton itself. For without commitment to change by all levels of management at the hospital the improvements we seek are unlikely to materialise in full measure.

I am proud as chairman to have been associated with the work of the Team. It has been a rewarding experience for us all. It only remains for me to record my personal thanks to Dr Julian Roberts who acted as chairman during the period of my absence in Southern Rhodesia as Election Commissioner.

Yours sincerely

Signed

JOHN BOYNTON

MEMBERS OF THE RAMPTON HOSPITAL MANAGEMENT REVIEW TEAM

SIR JOHN BOYNTON MC (CHAIRMAN): Formerly Chief Executive of Cheshire County Council. Company director and solicitor in private practice.

MRS M B ARMITAGE OBE BA (Admin): Formerly Director of Social Services, Sheffield.

CAPT W I DAVIES: Formerly a Prison Governor, member of the Prison Department Inspectorate and latterly Director of Prisons (Northern Ireland).

MRS C DERMODY SRN RNMS: A nursing sister at the Ellen Terry and Brooklands Unit, Queen Mary's Hospital, Carshalton, Surrey.

MR J C GARDNER SRN RNMS DHSA: Area Nursing Officer, Hertfordshire Area Health Authority.

MR D J KING BA AHA: District Administrator, Exeter Health Care District.

DR J M ROBERTS MD FRCPsych DPM: Consultant Psychiatrist, St. James' Hospital, Leeds and High Royds Hospital, Menston, and Senior Clinical Lecturer in Psychiatry, University of Leeds. Member of Yorkshire Regional Health Authority.

MR F WALTERS OBE JP FCA: Formerly Vice-Chairman of Trent Regional Health Authority.

DR C WILLIAMS MSc PhD: Principal Clinical Psychologist, Royal Western Counties Hospital, Exeter, Devon.

MR B WOOLLATT SRN RMN: Senior Charge Nurse, Drug Dependence Clinical Research and Treatment Unit, Bethlem Royal Hospital, Beckenham Kent.

Secretary: MR R M ORTON

Assistant Secretary (from 30.6.80): MR O C L THORPE

CONTENTS

PREFATORY NOTE: DEFINITION AND CLASSIFICATION OF MENTAL DISORDER

We refer in numerous places in our report to the different types of mental disorder which are statutorily recognised in the Mental Health Act 1959. It may be helpful to the reader to have set our here the text of the relevant subsections (4(1)–(4)) of the Act.

'4.—(1) In this Act "mental disorder" means mental illness, arrested or incomplete development of mind, psychopathic disorder, and any other disorder or disability of mind; and "mentally disordered" shall be construed accordingly.

(2) In this Act "severe subnormality" means a state of arrested or incomplete development of mind which includes subnormality of intelligence and is of such a nature or degree that the patient is incapable of living an independent life or of guarding himself against serious exploitation, or will be so incapable when of an age to do so.

(3) In this Act "subnormality" means a state of arrested or incomplete development of mind (not amounting to severe subnormality) which includes subnormality of intelligence and is of a nature or degree which requires or is susceptible to medical treatment or other special care or training of the patient.

(4) In this Act "psychopathic disorder" means a persistent disorder or disability of mind (whether or not including subnormality of intelligence) which results in abnormally aggressive or seriously irresponsible conduct on the part of the patient, and requires or is susceptible to medical treatment.'

It should be noted that the Act does not seek to define "mental illness".

Unless the reference is strictly to the legal definition, we generally follow normal current usage and employ the terms "mental handicap" and "severe mental handicap" in preference to "subnormality" and "severe subnormality".

LIST OF ABBREVIATIONS USED IN THIS REPORT

CNO   Chief Nursing Officer
DHSS   Department of Health and Social Security
DRO   Disablement Resettlement Officer
ECT   Electroconvulsive Therapy
EEG   Electro-encephalogram
GNC   General Nursing Council
HAS   Health Advisory Service
HDC   Heads of Departments Committee
HMT   Hospital Management Team
ITU   Industrial Training Unit
JCHPT   Joint Committee on Higher Psychiatric Training
MAC   Medical Advisory Committee
MHRT   Mental Health Review Tribunal
NHS   National Health Service
NO   Nursing Officer
PNO   Principal Nursing Officer
POA   Prison Officers' Association
PROPAR   Protection of Rights of Patients at Rampton
PSA   Property Services Agency of the Department of the Environment
RMN   Registered Mental Nurse
RMO   Responsible Medical Officer
RNMS   Registered Nurse for the Mentally Subnormal
RSU   Regional Secure Unit
SHOC   Special Hospitals Office Committee (of the Department of Health
          and Social Security)
SNO   Senior Nursing Officer
SRN   State Registered Nurse
UHF   Ultra High Frequency

CHAPTER 1

INTRODUCTION

1.1   On 15 May 1979 it became publicly known that Yorkshire Television had made a film about Rampton Hospital, one of the four 'special hospitals' run by the Department of Health and Social Security (DHSS) for persons detained under the Mental Health Act who in the opinion of the Secretary of State 'require treatment under conditions of special security on account of their dangerous, violent or criminal propensities'. The film, produced and directed by Mr John Willis and entitled 'The Secret Hospital', contained a large number of serious allegations of ill-treatment of patients by staff.

1.2   The film was shown on independent television on 22 May 1979. The Secretary of State for Social Services, Mr Patrick Jenkin MP, with senior DHSS officials had seen a preview on 17 May. On 21 May Mr Jenkin announced that he had referred the allegations of ill-treatment, many of which, if proved, would involve criminal assault, to the Director of Public Prosecutions who had arranged for a full investigation to be carried out by the Nottinghamshire police. He also announced that in the light of the allegations he had concluded that it was essential to institute a thorough review of the organisation and facilities at Rampton, including the monitoring of standards of care given, the procedure for dealing with complaints and the links which the hospital had with the outside world.

1.3   On 26 July Mr Jenkin announced the appointment of Sir John Boynton as the Chairman of what was to become known as the Rampton Hospital Management Review Team. He also announced the Team's terms of reference, which are set out in full in Appendix A. They required the Team 'to review the organisation, management and functioning of Rampton Special Hospital and to recommend changes where these are considered desirable', and specified particular aspects of Rampton's work which should be covered. The terms of reference made it clear that the Review should not in any way cut across the criminal investigations being carried out by the police for the Director of Public Prosecutions, and that it was not the function of the Review to collect or consider specific allegations of deliberate ill-treatment. If in the course of their work the Team came across evidence of such ill-treatment, they would be under a duty to transmit this evidence to the police unless it was clear that it had already been brought to their notice. The Team in fact—and this was perhaps to be expected—came across no evidence of ill-treatment of patients. They received only one letter containing fresh allegations of ill-treatment, from an ex-patient, which was referred to the police.

1.4   Following the appointment of the members of the Team we held our first meeting in London on 6 September 1979. Our next meeting was at Rampton from 16-19 October, when we had our first look round the hospital as a Team (although our Chairman had already visited the hospital twice since his appointment). We have since then had 14 further meetings of the Team as a whole, several of which have extended over more than one day.

1.5   But these formal meetings have constituted only a comparatively small part of our work. In terms of man-hours, the greatest part of our time has been spent actually looking at Rampton at work. For this purpose we divided ourselves at our meeting in October into seven working groups, dealing respectively with medical services; nursing services; social work and relations with the outside world; psychological services; education training and remedial therapy; administrative services; and management and organisation. Members of these groups have individually at various times spent several weeks at Rampton, observing all departments of the hospital at work, talking informally to staff and patients both individually and in groups, and examining documents and records. Members of the Team were issued with keys and were thus able to move freely and unannounced around the hospital; in fact they did so at all hours of the day and night. Nursing members in particular spent long hours on the wards over a period of nine weeks, and became sufficiently familiar figures to be able occasionally to assist directly in the care of patients. They were able to achieve a high level of understanding and in-depth knowledge of the everyday working of the hospital.

1.6   As well as talking to staff as we went round the hospital, we gave them the opportunity of expressing their views to us formally. We arranged for a 'suggestion form' to be distributed to all members of staff, together with a prepaid envelope addressed to our Chairman. Staff were assured of the absolute confidentiality of any information passed to the Team. They were also given the opportunity of asking for a private interview with a member of the Team if they wished. 59 completed forms were received, and 41 members of staff asked for and were given private interviews with members of the Team. The contents of the staff suggestion forms are summarised in Appendix B. We think the hospital ought to have a proper suggestion scheme. The suggestion box in the Lodge is not adequate for the purpose.

1.7   We did not undertake any corresponding exercise to seek comments from current or former patients at Rampton. It seemed to us that in view of the circumstances in which we were set up this would inevitably cause confusion between our role and that of the police who were investigating allegations of ill-treatment. We have however talked to a great many patients (and some visiting relatives) at Rampton. We also had a useful discussion with a small group of ex-patients and patients' relatives whose names were suggested to us as having information which would be relevant to our Review by Mr John Willis of Yorkshire Television and the organisation known as PROPAR (Protection of Rights of Patients At Rampton).

1.8   We wrote to a number of outside organisations whose views we thought would be helpful to our work. Most of them replied, in some cases with extremely full and carefully argued memoranda. A number of other organisations and individuals wrote to us, or, in some cases, asked to talk to us, and some further views sent initially to the DHSS were forwarded to us by them. We have carefully considered all this material, and are grateful to everyone who has taken the trouble to let us have their views. A list of organisations and individuals who gave their views to the Team is at Appendix C.

1.9   Soon after we had started work, the Parliamentary All Party Mental

Health Group under the Chairmanship of Mr Charles Irvine MP visited Rampton. They subsequently wrote to Mr Patrick Jenkin making a number of suggestions about Rampton. We were asked by DHSS Ministers to take account of these suggestions in the course of our work, and this we have done.

1.10   The Team, or individual members, have made visits to a number of other institutions, so that we could compare their problems with Rampton's and consider what lessons could be learned from their experience. In this country visits have been made to the other special hospitals (Broadmoor, Park Lane and Moss Side); the State Hospital at Carstairs in Scotland; the Eastdale Unit at Balderton Hospital, Newark; the interim secure unit at Rainhill Hospital, Merseyside; and Dartmoor, Exeter, Ford and Lincoln Prisons. We visited DHSS headquarters in London on several occasions. We also visited the Netherlands as we considered it essential to get an international perspective on the problems of dealing with dangerous psychiatric patients and it seemed to us from what we know of the Dutch approach to these problems that it would cast a particularly helpful light on policies and practices in this country. Members of the Team visited two institutions for mentally disordered offenders, the Hoeve Boschoord Clinic near Steenwijk and the Van der Hoeven Clinic at Utrecht; mental handicap hospitals at Nordwijk and Venray; the forensic psychiatry unit at the State Mental Hospital at Eindhoven; and the Selection Institute and the Psychiatric Observation Clinic, both at Utrecht. Our observations there reinforced our intention to follow up a number of lines of approach which we were tentatively considering prior to our departure.

1.11   The Team asked three specialist 'assessors' to advise them on particular aspects of Rampton's work. We were advised on nurse education by Mr S J Holder SRN STD RNT DipEd (London) FRCN, Director of Nurse Education at St Mary's Hospital, Paddington; on the patients' school by Mr C A Norman, formerly Her Majesty's Inspector (Staff Inspector) at the Department of Education and Science; and on dental services by Mr G V Morrell LDS, Area Dental Officer, Leeds Area Health Authority (Teaching). We wish to express our gratitude to all three assessors for their invaluable help and advice. We have not however asked them to sign this report, and we alone take responsibility for its contents.

1.12   We have not seen our role primarily as that of sitting in judgment on Rampton and attributing praise and blame, but rather of providing help and advice to enable Rampton to become a better place for patients and staff. For this reason we have aimed to work in as open a way as possible and to secure the agreement of staff and management to our proposals in the course of our work, rather than to unveil in our final report a long list of hitherto undisclosed recommendations. The Team as a whole spent three days in July 1980 discussing the most important of our provisional conclusions and recommendations with management and staff representatives at Rampton. The atmosphere at these meetings was in general helpful and constructive, and we found them of great assistance in formulating our recommendations in their final form. We were able at a subsequent meeting in September to obtain a commitment from the staff to the early implementation of some of our more straightforward recommendations, for example some of those concerning the

3

quality of life on the male block wards, and we are pleased to record that a number of these recommendations have already been implemented. What is more important, staff are examining their own attitudes and philosophies of treatment and there is some indication that the 'institutional inertia' to which we refer more than once in this report, is already beginning to be recognised and challenged.

1.13   We would like to express our thanks to all those at Rampton and the DHSS who have helped us in our work. At the best of times a review of this sort would have put a great additional burden on the shoulders of Rampton staff at all levels. In our case we were very conscious that we were descending on the hospital at a time when the staff felt very much under threat in the light of the Yorkshire Television programme, the subsequent publicity and the police enquiries (which have continued throughout most of the period of our work). We would therefore like to pay tribute here to the helpful, patient and efficient way in which both at Rampton and DHSS, staff have at this very difficult time coped with all our various demands and answered our queries. They have made our task a great deal easier than it might otherwise have been.

1.14   We have written our report in two parts. In Part I we have tried to introduce the reader to the background of our work, to set our conclusions in their wider context, and to give a general account of our principal conclusions and recommendations. Part II considers the various aspects of the work of the hospital in more detail. This distinction between Parts I and II should not however be taken to imply that all the important material in our report is contained in Part I. In both Part I and Part II we make recommendations and suggestions as we go along, but we also list them separately at the end of our report.

PART I

CHAPTER 2

RAMPTON: THE GENERAL BACKGROUND

2.1 The Special Hospitals

2.1.1 Under the Mental Health Act 1959, the Minister of Health was required to provide 'special hospitals', defined as institutions for persons subject to detention under the Act who in the Minister's opinion 'require treatment under conditions of special security on account of their dangerous, violent or criminal propensities'. This provision was subsequently re-enacted in National Health Service (NHS) legislation, and is now to be found, with references to 'the Secretary of State' substituted for those to the 'Minister of Health' in Section 4 of the NHS Act 1977.

2.1.2 There are four special hospitals in England and Wales—Broadmoor, Rampton, Moss Side and Park Lane. The title 'special hospital' itself dates only from the 1959 Act, but three of the four hospitals—Broadmoor, Rampton and Moss Side—were already in existence when the Act came into force.

    a. *Broadmoor Hospital* (at Crowthorn, three miles south of Bracknell in Berkshire), the oldest, was opened in 1863 as a criminal lunatic asylum run by the Home Office. No one could be sent to Broadmoor unless he had been charged before a court. Mentally handicapped patients, whether offenders or not, could not be admitted. In 1949 the ownership of Broadmoor was transferred from the Home Office to the Ministry of Health, and its management taken over by the Board of Control.

    b. *Rampton Hospital* the next oldest, began life in 1912 as a criminal lunatic asylum like Broadmoor. In 1919 however, responsibility for it was transferred from the Home Office to the Board of Control, and it took on a new role in 1920 as a state institution for 'mental defectives with dangerous and violent propensities', run by the Board of Control. It admitted only mentally handicapped people, those who had been found guilty by the courts of an offence and those who had been detained in hospital under the ordinary compulsory provisions of the Mental Deficiency Act but who had dangerous and violent propensities. In 1947 ownership was transferred to the Minister of Health under the provisions of the NHS Act, but the hospital continued to be managed by the Board of Control.

    c. *Moss Side Hospital* (at Maghull, nine miles north of Liverpool) was opened in 1919 as a state institution for mental defectives, like Rampton. (It was however not used as such between 1920 and 1933, when it was leased to the Ministry of Pensions for use as an epileptic colony.) Like Rampton, it was transferred to the Minister of Health in 1947, and was managed by the Board of Control.

    d. *Park Lane Hospital* (on a site adjacent to Moss Side) is still under construction—an 'advance unit' opened in 1979.

2.1.3 The Board of Control was abolished by the 1959 Act, and the existing special hospitals were brought under direct control of the Minister of Health (later the Secretary of State for Social Services). The Act contained a specific bar on special hospitals being administered as part of the NHS by local hospital authorities (though this was later removed, by the NHS reorganisation Act 1973). The Act also had the effect of making it legally possible for any patient needing treatment in a special hospital to be admitted to any of the three hospitals then existing, whether or not they have been before a court, and whatever their Mental Health Act classification (mental illness, psycho-pathic disorder, subnormality, severe subnormality—see the Prefatory Note to our report).

2.1.4   The Secretary of State controls all admissions to special hospitals. Although in theory, as indicated above, any patient can be admitted to any one of the four hospitals, in practice virtually all mentally handicapped patients still go to Rampton or Moss Side. Most of the more intelligent mentally ill and psychopathic patients go to Broadmoor or Park Lane; the less intelligent go to Rampton or Moss Side. It follows from the policies we have outlined that Rampton serves patients coming from the whole of England and Wales, and not those coming from any particular geographical area.

2.2   The function of special hospitals

2.2.1   The present statutory basis for the provision of special hospitals does not say explicitly what the specific functions of special hospitals should be. To attempt to analyse those functions in any detail would be to go beyond our terms of reference, and would raise wide issues, many of them extremely difficult and controversial, about the way in which mentally disordered people, who include mentally disordered offenders, are treated in our society. Any wider review of the special hospitals as a whole, such as that which we suggest in Chapter 4, would need to look at these issues in detail. But we are nevertheless obliged to say something ourselves on the subject of Rampton's aims and objectives as we can hardly comment on Rampton's 'management, organisation and functioning' without some preliminary consideration of the role the hospital is meant to be fulfilling.

2.2.2   The statute makes it clear that special hospitals are intended to provide at any rate two things: 'treatment' and 'conditions of special security'. We take 'security' in the context of a psychiatric hospital to mean arrangements designed to prevent compulsorily detained patients (a) from leaving the hospital in which they are being treated except with the consent of and on such conditions as those responsible for their treatment may wish to lay down and (b) from causing harm to themselves, other patients or staff. 'Special security' we take to imply that in special hospitals it is intended that relatively more resources will be devoted to security than in other psychiatric hospitals.

2.2.3   The reason why the patients for whom special hospitals are intended need conditions of 'special security' is, according to the statute, because of their 'dangerous, violent or criminal propensities'. However that formula is to be interpreted, we think it is clear that the aim of security at special hospitals should be protection, primarily of the public but also of the patient himself, other patients and the staff. Special hospitals differ from prisons in this regard. Prisons deprive people of their liberty primarily as a punishment. We accept of course that the need to protect the public is a factor which a court may take into account when fixing the length of a prison sentence. However, when making a hospital order under the Mental Health Act the court has no power to fix a period of detention. The protection of the public is a matter which has to be considered by those responsible for considering the discharge or transfer of any patient from a special hospital. The absence of provision for any fixed period of detention in a special hospital reinforces our view that the concept of paying a penalty for an offence should have no place in the philosophy of the special hospitals. We have found nothing in legislation or elsewhere which suggests that special hospitals should have any such penal function. Such a function would in any case in our view be inconsistent with the idea of a hospital. As our report will make clear however this principle is not always reflected in the actual regime at Rampton.

2.2.4   The other function of special hospitals is to provide 'treatment'. Section 147(1) of the Mental Health Act says that 'medical treatment' should be interpreted as including nursing and also 'care and training under medical supervision'. On this basis 'treatment' need not be directed towards a cure or indeed an amelioration of a patient's illness; it could just be looking after him. But we see no reason to be pessimistic about the susceptibility to active treatment of the majority of patients in Rampton or the likelihood of a successful outcome. Most Rampton patients eventually become fit to leave and indeed Rampton discharges more patients in proportion to its population than the other special hospitals. We draw attention here to the policy document entitled 'The aims of Rampton Hospital' which was produced by the then Hospital Committee at Rampton in 1972 and which we reproduce at Appendix D. This is the nearest thing to an 'official' statement of Rampton's treatment aims. According to this document the primary purpose of the hospital's work, apart from its security function, should be 'to prepare patients for return to the community as soon as possible'. It recognises that the ultimate goal of preparing a patient to a level where he can return to and survive in the community is an ideal which may, in practice, be difficult to achieve, but it is urged that thsese difficulties should not be viewed as insurmountable. Many patients will of course not be able to go directly from Rampton to living in the community. For the majority the 'next stop' will be a NHS psychiatric hospital. But subject to that proviso, the treatment aims set out in the 1972 document are ones which we would wholeheartedly endorse.

2.2.5   The two functions of a special hospital—security and treatment—can often conflict; what is good from the point of view of treatment may be bad from the point of view of security. We discuss this further in Chapters 8 and 18; all we would say here is that we think the conflict when it arises is a genuine one which can be tackled only on the basis of compromise and the balance of probabilities.

2.3   Rampton's site and buildings

2.3.1   Rampton Hospital is situated in north Nottinghamshire in the middle of a gently rolling and uneventful agricultural landscape in which the cooling towers of West Burton, Cottam and High Marnham power stations a few miles away on the Trent feature prominently. The hospital has its own estate of 185 staff houses just outside the security perimeter; otherwise the nearest

8

settlement is Rampton village, about a mile and a half away. The nearest town is Retford, six miles away, where many of the staff live; it has a population of 18,000. Of larger centres of population, Lincoln is about 16 miles away, Newark 17, Doncaster 25 and Sheffield and Nottingham each about 33. The geographical situation of the hospital can thus fairly be described as remote.

2.3.2   The original hospital buildings were completed in 1912, and although there have been considerable additions since, their outward appearance has remained substantially unaltered since that date. There is a central high security area (with exercise areas) chiefly comprising five three-storeyed blocks of wards, plus workshops, the patients' education centre, the chapel and gymnasium (both modern), and administration and other offices, linked together by long corridors. This inner area is surrounded by an 18 foot concrete wall. Outside the wall is a comparatively less secure area, surrounded by a sunken wall and ditch, within which is a 17 foot high chainlink fence. In this area are detached two-storey 'villa' wards, mostly built between the wars, for pre-release and less dangerous patients, with a football pitch and sports field. This area is floodlit at night, to allow patients to be moved safely from building to building. Outside the secure area altogether are the staff housing estate and nurses' residences, the School of Nursing, the staff canteen, club and playing fields, most doctors' offices and the hospital social work and finance departments. There is also a hospital farm and market garden of 60 acres.

2.4   The Rampton patients

2.4.1   Rampton's official bed complement is 1,070, but its present patient population (30 June 1980) is 814, 622 men and 192 women. There are marked differences between the male and female populations.

2.4.2   Under the Mental Health Act 1959 patients are classified under four diagnostic categories, mental illness, psychopathic disorder, subnormality and severe subnormality (see the Prefatory Note to our report). The percentage of male patients at Rampton with a principal classification under each category is as follows:

Mental Illness	40%
Psychopathic disorder	28%
Subnormality or severe subnormality	32%

2.4.3   It should be borne in mind that many patients have a multiple diagnosis and that as a result of the DHSS admission policy (see paragraph 2.1.4), the intelligence of those classified as mentally ill or suffering from psychopathic disorder is often well below average and in many cases bordering on the mentally handicapped level. About 75 per cent of male patients come to Rampton from the courts, ie they have committed offences, and just over 60 per cent are 'restricted', ie they cannot be discharged or transferred without the consent of the Home Secretary (see paragraph 9.1.2(a)). About 80 per cent of the male population of Rampton in 1979 had been in Rampton less than ten years, compared with about 75 per cent in 1970.

2.4.4   Amongst the female patients at Rampton, on the other hand, principal classifications are distributed as follows:

9

Mental illness	23%
Psychopathic disorder	19%
Subnormality or severe subnormality (severe subnormality 46%)	58%

2.4.5   Only about 25 per cent of the women are offenders and fewer than that 'restricted'. Only 58 per cent of the female patients have been resident for less than ten years in 1979, (66 per cent in 1970). These relatively long stays reflect the preponderance of mentally handicapped patients among the female population.

2.4.6   Rampton's patient population is a young one. Two-thirds are under 40, and only 2 per cent over 60. There is a turnover in the population of about 15 per cent per year; latterly about 70-80 patients a year have transferred to NHS hospitals and about 40-50 have been discharged directly to the community.

2.4.7   Rampton's reducing patient numbers (1,080 in 1973, 814 now) and changing patient mix (50 per cent classified as subnormal or severely subnormal in 1974, 40 per cent now) reflect a changing pattern of applications and perhaps some change of emphasis in the policies of the DHSS who control special hospital admissions. Fewer patients are being accepted for the special hospitals (about 200 a year now compared with 350 in the early seventies). The Mental Health Act classifications of the patients accepted over the past three years have been:

Mentally ill	60%
Psychopathic disorder	20%
Subnormal	16%
Severely subnormal	4%

If present trends continue, we can foresee a time in the mid eighties when the hospital will have fewer than 700 patients of which only a quarter will be mentally handicapped. This would have substantial implications for Rampton's future which we discuss in paragraphs 5.10 and 5.11.

2.4.8   A more detailed stastical account of Rampton's patient population is at Appendix E.

2.5   The Wards

2.5.1   When patients are first admitted to Rampton, they normally spend four to six months on an admission ward in the inner high security area of the hospital. They are then normally allocated to one of the other block wards, where they may spend two or three years. They can then move to a villa ward in the outer medium security area. After a period in the villas, most patients, given satisfactory progress, can be expected to be transferred to a NHS hospital or to be discharged. All wards are single sex: practices, style and attitudes vary considerably between the male and female sides of the hospital which are for many purposes run quite separately.

2.6 The Rampton staff

2.6.1 There were 935 staff (whole-time equivalent) employed by DHSS in post at Rampton on 30 June 1980. They were made up as follows:

Doctors	16	(plus one part-timer)
Nurses	611	
Social workers	10	
Psychologists	2	
Occupations staff	89	
Administrative staff (including secretaries and typists)	49	
Church of England Chaplain	1	
Ancillary and other staff	157	

In addition there were 11 teachers and a librarian who are employed by the Nottinghamshire County Council, but whose salaries are largely reimbursed by DHSS, a hospital pharmacist and technician employed by the Nottingham Area Health Authority (Teaching), and 90 maintenance and engineering staff (not exclusively employed at Rampton—see paragraph 28.4) employed by the Property Services Agency (PSA) of the Department of the Environment.

2.6.2 Except for those employed by the local authority, the hospital staff are civil servants. Different groups of staff are however paid on different bases and have different terms and conditions of service. Doctors, nurses, psychologists and ancillary staff are in practice paid on the same scales as NHS staff (plus the special hospitals lead—see the next paragraph). Occupations staff are in grades peculiar to the special hospitals: their pay is linked with that of the nurses. Social workers' pay and conditions are roughly based on those of local authority social workers, but the position is rather complicated—see paragraph 26.5.2. The administrative staff are in ordinary civil service grades.

2.6.3 Most staff receive a special pay lead over normal NHS pay rates, common to all special hospitals. It is currently £926 a year for doctors, nurses, occupations staff and others in direct charge of patients. Other grades whose duties may involve close contact with patients receive half lead. The lead was first introduced in 1923 for nurses at Broadmoor and later for nurses at Rampton and Moss Side. It is intended to take account of the differences between the working conditions of special hospital staff and those of staff in other psychiatric hospitals.

2.6.4 For historical reasons the trades union to which most of the nursing, occupations and ancillary staff at Rampton belong is the Prison Officers' Association (POA). The POA is the only union represented on the staff side of the local Whitley Committee.

11

CHAPTER 3

EARLIER REPORTS ON RAMPTON

3.1   We are not the first body in recent years to have investigated Rampton. We think it is worth referring briefly to some earlier investigations and their outcome.

3.2   The last comprehensive look at the special hospitals as a whole was by the House of Commons Estimates Committee in 1967–68.* The Committee made a number of detailed recommendations but, with some reservations as to Broadmoor, found that the special hospitals were 'performing more than satisfactorily the functions Parliament entrusted to them'.

3.3   In 1971 a team from the Hospital Advisory Service (HAS: now the Health Advisory Service) spent a fortnight at Rampton on a routine visit, and produced a confidential report to the then Secretary of State, which the DHSS and the current Director of the HAS agreed could be made available to us. They made over 60 recommendations, many quite detailed. A number of these, notably those commending a more multi-disciplinary style of management, with a system of clinical teams and multi-disciplinary case conferences (see paragraphs 7.4 and 29.2.7) have subsequently been implemented. Little progress has been made on others, notably those recommending a change in the nursing shift system (see Chapter 10) and the introduction of joint medical appointments with appropriate outside psychiatric services (see paragraph 16.2.5). But many of these recommendations were subsequently overtaken by the Elliott Report—see next paragraph.

3.4   The next and, before we were appointed, the last detailed look at Rampton was by Mr James Elliott in 1973. Mr Elliott had been a hospital administrator and was at that time an Associate Director of the King's Fund. He was appointed by the DHSS in the aftermath of an abortive attempt by them to modify the existing shift system for nurses, as recommended by the HAS, which had led to industrial action by the nursing staff. His remit was to look at organisational problems, and staff management relationships at Rampton. Mr Elliott spent three weeks at Rampton interviewing staff and observing the work of the hospital. His report to the Secretary of State was again confidential, but seems to have been widely leaked. The report which was made available to us by DHSS, is difficult to summarise briefly. It pointed to the need for some fundamental changes of attitude within the hospital, and made some specific recommendations, listed in Appendix F, with most of which, as will subsequently be made clear, we are basically in sympathy. There has, however, been only limited progress in implementing the more important recommendations.

3.5   It is probably fair to say that our review has not come up with any startling new truths about Rampton. It is also fair to say that it has been more thorough than any of its predecessors, both in terms of man-hours spent

---

*Second Report, Session 1967–68. The Special Hospitals and the State Hospital. HMSO March 1968.

observing the work of the hospital and in the breadth of the context in which we have endeavoured to consider its problems. We are confident that we have spent long enough at Rampton for us to get below the surface and to see it as it really is, both in its strengths and its weaknesses. It is in the light of that that we hope that our recommendations will be considered.

CHAPTER 4

THE WIDER CONTEXT OF OUR REVIEW

4.1 Our terms of reference required us to look at the problems of Rampton, rather than to consider suggestions about the future of the special hospitals generally. Nevertheless in the course of our work on Rampton we have been made aware of a number of radical suggestions, some of which have been the subject of public discussion in recent years. One is that the present four special hospitals should in the long term be replaced by a much larger number of smaller regionally based units. Another is that special hospitals should be retained, but should be run as part of the regional structure of the NHS, as recommended by the 'Three Chairmen's Enquiry' in 1976.* A less radical version of this suggestion is that the special hospitals should be run more or less as at present, but that their catchment areas should be 'regionalised'. We have become conscious that the role of all the special hospitals is in any event being affected, and will be affected in the future (in a way which it is impossible at this time to predict with any degree of certainty) by two important current developments. One is the changing pattern of admissions to special hospitals, to which we referred in paragraph 2.4.6 and which reflects changing ideas about the treatment and care of patients with 'dangerous violent or criminal propensities'. The other is the proposed programme of NHS regional secure units which has as yet barely got off the ground.

4.2 We have not considered these matters in any detail, as they are outside our terms of reference and go beyond the immediate problems of Rampton, (although we recognise that regionalisation of catchment areas and some form of integration with the NHS would make a number of Rampton's problems easier to solve). But we think that the issues raised are sufficiently interesting and important for the DHSS to consider whether a wider review of the future role of the special hospitals is called for, the sort of review which we ourselves are not constituted to undertake, even if it fell within our terms of reference. We note that the last general review of the special hospitals was the Estimates Committee investigation in 1967/68 (see paragraph 3.2 above).

4.3 The suggestion has been put to us in the course of our review that a commitment should be made now to closing Rampton and replacing it with new, smaller, regionally based units close to centres of population, medical schools and other hospitals. This suggestion would ideally best be considered in the context of a wider review such as that we have suggested. Nevertheless, to the extent that the suggestion is specifically related to Rampton, we have thought it right to express our own views on it, basing those views on what we have learned at Rampton rather than on wider considerations.

4.4 The argument for closing Rampton runs briefly as follows. Rampton's problems arise primarily because, compared even with the other special hospitals, it is too isolated, geographically, organisationally and professionally,

---

*Regional Chairmen's Enquiry into the working of the DHSS in relation to Regional Health Authorities. A Report by the Chairmen of the Regional Health Authorities of the National Health Service. Reproduced by the Department of Health and Social Security, May 1976.

and because it is too big. This isolation, the argument continues, is a necessary corollary of its geographical position, which effectively prevents it from forming close and continuing links with universities, medical schools and other hospitals and from attracting good quality professional staff from outside. One of the reasons why it is too big is that it has a nation-wide catchment area, and this in turn contributes to its organisational isolation, by making it difficult to run it as part of the regional structure of the NHS. It is argued that Rampton's past history shows that neither exhortation and encouragement nor changes in the managerial structure have succeeded in overcoming institutional inertia and bringing about the 'attitudinal swings' which are necessary if the hospital is to function to an acceptable standard. From this it is inferred that our own recommendations are unlikely to fare any better; Rampton's size and isolation, entrenched staff attitudes at all levels, and all the resulting sociological pressures in favour of the status quo will effectively neutralise them. So the only answer, the argument concludes, is to give Rampton up as a bad job, and replace it by new institutions which can start off without Rampton's inherent disadvantages.

4.5   As a diagnosis of some of Rampton's principal problems, there is much in the above with which we agree. As paragraph 5.11 will make clear, we agree that Rampton's patient population is too big, and we think that it ought to be made smaller. We also agree that many of Rampton's problems stem from its isolation, geographical and otherwise. But we do not agree that the right answer to these problems is to close Rampton. In practice of course Rampton could not be closed overnight or anything approaching it: it would have to be phased out over a period whilst alternative facilities were being planned and provided, much as Park Lane is being developed to reduce the size of Broadmoor. The evidence of the Park Lane project suggests that to plan and build replacements for Rampton would take many years. During this period of 'blight', morale at Rampton would be bound to be very seriously affected and in our view there would be very little chance of many of our recommendations for significant improvements in regime, treatment and so on being implemented. All Rampton's existing faults would be perpetuated for, we would guess, at the very least another ten years, and this could have a very damaging effect on patients. We do not think we would be justified in making any recommendations which would have such an effect unless we thought that Rampton's prognosis was hopeless and that this sort of lingering euthanasia was the only solution.

4.6   We are very far from taking this view. We have found much that is good at Rampton. Many excellent staff are providing their patients with care, development and training of a high standard in an environment in many ways superior of that of NHS psychiatric hospitals. The standard of nursing care on the female block wards and on the villa wards is generally good, and we admired very much the painstaking and dedicated work of nurses from the Activity Group in organising social and sporting activities for all patients as well as running specialised activities of various sorts for the more severely disturbed or handicapped patients. Many NHS hospitals could learn much from Rampton's School of Nursing, patients' education department and occupations department. We have been impressed by the hospital's ability to

15

maintain good staffing levels at a time when some other special hospitals are having difficulties in this sphere, and to provide patients with a high degree of personal supervision. We have noted that each year Rampton discharges and transfers a higher proportion of its patient population than the other special hospitals. The standards of maintenance and decorative order of the buildings are in general admirable. We are convinced that given a sufficient degree of commitment by all concerned these and other good features can be built on and that the changes and improvements needed at Rampton can be achieved. We do not therefore believe that the hospital should be closed. But having said that, we would not rule out as a possible option for consideration in a wider and longer term review the replacement of all the special hospitals by a number of smaller units providing a service for a NHS region or group of regions.

4.7   There is one other wider issue, with implications extending well beyond the special hospitals, which it seems appropriate to mention in this chapter. At present there is no mechanism, as in local authority institutions, NHS hospitals and prisons, to ensure a regular and authorised public scrutiny of the special hospitals. Neither Regional nor Area Health Authorities are involved with Rampton, nor is the requirement met by the large number of people visiting the hospital on official parties (although such visits are valuable to Rampton—see paragraph 31.5.2). Visitors of this sort are guests on guided tours and do not fulfil the function of public watchdog. DHSS officials are in no position to make frequent ward visits and talk to the staff and patients, and in any case they cannot be expected to act both as servants of the Secretary of State and representatives of the public. Although Community Health Councils (CHCs) have recently been invited to visit Rampton and the other special hospitals, and in fact have done so, they have no formal powers. Mental Health Review Tribunals (MHRTs) have an important function in considering whether patients should continue to be detained under the Mental Health Act, but have no powers to investigate complaints or to comment on treatment or standards of care. The visits of the HAS are infrequent and are undertaken by different teams on different occasions; their reports are advisory and as a rule confidential, and do not have any more formal backing. We think that on the face of it there is a strong case for an appointed body to inspect and monitor closed institutions such as Rampton and the other special hospitals, or indeed wherever patients are subject to detention under the Mental Health Act. The exact powers and functions of such a body would be for further consideration, but we think it might be constituted on the lines of the old Board of Control or the Scottish Mental Welfare Commission. Its functions might include the review of patient care and treatment, the independent investigation of more serious complaints (from whatever source) and a general protective function on behalf of detained patients which need not necessarily cut across the functions of MHRTs. Such a protective function might include some responsibilities in connection with the difficult problem of consent to treatment in respect of detained patients, some 60 per cent of whom reside in the Special Hospitals. We commend this idea to the Secretary of State for fuirther detailed consideration and discussion with interested bodies. If our proposals for a Review Board for Rampton (see Chapter 6) are accepted, we visualise the Board as carrying out a degree of public surveillance of Rampton,

16

but the point we are making applies to all places where patients are compulsorily detained, not just to Rampton itself.

CHAPTER 5

KEY ISSUES AND KEY RECOMMENDATIONS

5.1   In this chapter we summarise our diagnosis of Rampton's ills and indicate the general lines of our prescription for putting them right. Of its nature this chapter concentrates on Rampton's shortcomings, and taken in isolation paints a one-sided picture. As we explained in paragraph 4.6 above, we have found much that is good at Rampton; we gave some examples in that paragraph, and there will be more later in our report. Moreover we think our criticisms of Rampton must be placed firmly in the context of the exceptionally difficult job which society has given the staff of the special hospitals to do. Caring for the sort of patients who are admitted to Rampton can be arduous and unrewarding, and is sometimes dangerous. It is vital not to underestimate the amount of professional dedication and sheer hard work expected from staff at Rampton day in and day out. But there are things which are wrong at Rampton and it will take a sustained and purposeful effort by all concerned if they are to be put right.

5.2   Professional leadership

5.2.1   In general, the order in which we list Rampton's shortcomings in this chapter should not be taken as reflecting the relative importance we ascribe to them. Nevertheless, we think that it is right to mention lack of professional leadership as the first item on the list, because in our view this deficiency has made a very large contribution to Rampton's problems. We are thinking here primarily of the medical profession. The low level of medical participation in the general management of the hospital, which we discuss further in Chapter 16, has been one feature of this lack of leadership. We recognise that the way clinical work has been distributed between the consultant staff has not made it easy for particular consultants to devote a lot of time to management. We also recognise that there have been encouraging signs of improvement in this areas since our appointment. But we also think that doctors could reasonably have been expected to provide non-medical staff in the wards and departments with leadership and guidance on a day-to-day basis in matters of treatment and care. In general, although there have of course been notable exceptions, we do not think this has been forthcoming. We are not however criticising the medical staff alone. We believe the standard of professional leadership amongst the Rampton nurse managers has fallen below the standard we think it is reasonable to expect. One of the effects of this lack of professional leadership has been that the challenge and opportunities for the application of modern psychiatric nursing techniques have not been fully seized. We are criticising here not so much individuals, who we think have in general done their best in unpromising circumstances, as a system which has not allowed proper leadership to emerge.

5.2.2   To some extent, not surprisingly, the local officials of the Prison Officers' Association have filled the 'leadership vacuum' at Rampton. No doubt reflecting the views of their members, they have been unenthusiastic in the past about some desirable changes and to that extent must take some responsibility for Rampton's continuing problems. This is not to deny that the

18

staff have made suggestions for change and improvement over the years. Changes have taken place and there have been improvements. The way Rampton has been managed however has made it difficult for ideas for change to be implemented.

5.2.3   It is largely to combat this lack of professional leadership that we think a Medical Director should be appointed for Rampton. He would have the job of co-ordinating the medical work of the hospital and would provide co-ordination and leadership for the hospital as a whole. We elaborate on this further in chapter 6, but would make it clear that we are not contemplating an autocratic appointment like that held by former Medical Superintendents, but the appointment of a leader of the Hospital Mangement Team, with as much emphasis on the team as on its leader.

5.3   Ward regimes and patients' quality of life

5.3.1   Rampton is a large and complex institution, and what is true of one clinical area, ward, department or even nursing shift may well not be true of another. Generalisations about nursing practices in different parts of the hospital must therefore be made with caution. Nevertheless we think it is fair to say that on the male block wards (we exempt the female wards and the male villas from much of this criticism) we have found in general a tradition of inflexible and over-structured regimes, with too much insistence on conformity to rigid disciplinary rules and too little scope for the development by patients of self-awareness and self-control. We accept that in any large institution everyday life must in practice to some extent be governed by rules and regulations to which everyone must be subject. We also accept that in the special circumstances of Rampton, a proper degree of discipline and routine is necessary if internal security is to be safeguarded. Nevertheless we think that in general security is too often used indiscriminately at Rampton as a 'catch all' excuse for resisting many measures which would give a better quality of life to patients and improve their therapeutic environment. There should be a minimum standard which should reflect current perceptions of what is reasonable. No agreed standard exists at present and practice sets the threshold at too low a level.

5.3.2   We give a detailed account of life on the male block wards in the Annex to Part I of our report, and list in Chapter 11 a number of specific examples of the sort of features which we find objectionable. We give just one example here, by way of illustration; we are glad to say that since this part of our report was disclosed to and discussed with management and staff, steps have already been taken to reconsider and amend the practice existing up to August 1980. This was that patients were as a universal practice not allowed to use a transistor radio and, in the male block wards, patients were not allowed to have furniture, other than a bed, pictures or personal possessions in their rooms. The bare and spartan standard of comfort, personalisation and amenity was particularly unfortunate in a regime where nearly half the day has to be spent locked in such a room. We think in respects such as this the quality of life in the male block wards falls below acceptable standards, and recommend that changes should be made accordingly. As we have said, some changes have been made and others are under consideration.

19

5.4 The organisation of the patients' day

There is another respect in which we think patients' quality of life should be improved, and this affects all patients, not just those on the male block wards. We think it is wholly unacceptable for patients to be confined to their bedrooms for about 11 hours or more each night, for evening activities to be as restricted as they are and for the active day (particularly for those patients who attend the school) to be kept as short as it is. What may have had some justification as a routine for severely mentally handicapped patients seems to us increasingly inappropriate for the different kind of patients who now predominate in the patient population. All these features of patients' life seem to a large extent to be effects of the present nursing shift system, and we recommend in Chapter 10 that consultations should begin with the staff to review it. We recognise that changes in the shift system would have far-reaching implications for staff's daily life.

5.5 Treatment programmes

It is not only patients' quality of life which we think is adversely affected by the regime on the block wards. We also think it results in too much rigidity and inflexibility in treatment programmes. We do not think that the undoubted need for orderly routines on the wards should preclude each patient having an individual treatment programme designed in the light of a multi-disciplinary assessment of his or her needs and potentialities. If this aim is to be achieved however we recognise that present staffing levels may need to be reviewed. We discuss this further in Chapter 7. It should amongst other things involve the provision of much better facilities for individual interviews with patients in rooms set aside for this purpose (see paragraph 11.1.3). There would also have to be a much greater input from clinical psychologists, who have been in chronically short supply at Rampton for many years. We recommend that for this and other reasons every effort must be made to recruit an adequate number of psychologists at the hospital (see Chapter 25).

5.6 Integration of the sexes

We think that a careful extension of integration of the sexes, both of staff and patients, would be an important contribution towards a more flexible therapeutic approach. There is some limited mixing of the sexes now, on social occasions and at other times, but we think there should be more opportunities for patients, particularly those with sexual and other emotional problems, to learn in an everyday context how to relate better socially to people of the opposite sex. We fully understand the misgivings which some Rampton staff have expressed about further integration. However, we did see such integration working successfully in institutions in Holland. We think some of the occupations workshops might be the best place at Rampton for further experiments in this area. This is discussed further in paragraphs 7.3.4-5 and 23.4.3.

5.7 The security regime in the villas

Another area where we think greater flexibility should be possible is in the security regime for pre-release patients in the villa areas. We elaborate on this in Chapter 8. In brief, and without wishing to minimise the problems, we consider that more could be done to provide pre-discharge patients with conditions more nearly approximating to those in the community to which they will be returning.

5.8 Nursing staff uniforms

We believe that the present prison officer style uniform worn by the male-nursing staff gives an inappropriate and unhelpful symbolic expression to the custodial aspects to their role. We recognise that there are good security grounds for keeping a distinctive uniform of some sort for nurses but we think that the style of the uniform should be changed to something more appropriate to a therapeutic environment. We discuss general questions of nursing 'style' further in Chapter 18.

5.9 Rampton's isolation

5.9.1 We think that Rampton suffers seriously from its isolation —geographical, organisational, professional and social. The geographical isolation creates tremendous difficulties for patients' relatives, as we explain further in paragraph 31.3.4–7, and we think their needs should be given much more attention. They should be given more information about how Rampton works and how they can find out about patients' progress. Visiting arrangements should be improved. In particular visiting on the male villas should be reintroduced and this facility should also be available on all the female villas. The possible demand for catering, accommodation or creche facilities by visitors should be investigated, and visitors who travel by private car, as well as though using public transport, should be eligible for assistance with travelling expenses.

5.9.2 Rampton's professional and social isolation have produced what we think is in many ways an inbred and inward-looking community, and has helped to perpetuate old-fashioned staff attitudes. We think an important contribution towards breaking down this isolation could be made by re-negotiating the national agreement on promotion of nurses in special hospitals so as to allow recruitment of nurses from outside Rampton at charge nurse and nursing officer level. Training (see next paragraph) will also have a key role in this area. In particular, since many staff in post have little experience outside Rampton, we think it is particularly important that they should be given secondments visits and attachments to gain first hand experience of alternative approaches to psychiatric care. We think there is also a case for encouraging distinguished representatives of the health professions and also research workers to come to work at Rampton for periods of time. We discuss these issues further in paragraph 18.4.3–4

5.10 Staff education and training

We think there should be a radical review of the education and training needs of all staff at Rampton. This has become particularly urgent because of recent changes in Rampton's patient mix (see paragraph 2.4.6). Only a third of the patients are now legally classified as mentally handicapped, and we think the proportion will and should continue to fall. We do not think that *severely* mentally handicapped patients should in fact be admitted to special

21

hospitals at all other than in exceptional circumstances. But in many ways the hospital is still run as a hospital exclusively for the mentally handicapped. Although we are convinced that it is essential that the School of Nursing at Rampton should continue, and that it has a vital role in maintaining standards of patient care and ensuring adequate recruitment of staff, we recognise that recent changes in patient mix have made mental handicap training less appropriate. In any case the specialised nature of experience available in a special hospital creates difficulties for basic training, whether in mental handicap or mental illness. In Chapter 19 we invite the General Nursing Council (GNC) to consider at their forthcoming visit to Rampton what sort of courses, basic and post-qualification, the School of Nursing should in future be offering. We also believe (see Chapter 20) that there should be a major increase in the resources devoted to in-service training and secondments for all staff and that consideration should be given to setting up a united in-service training department for all diciplines at the hospital.

5.11   Number of patients

We believe that Rampton's patient population is still too large, even though it has beeen falling steadily since 1973 (see paragraph 2.4.6). We would deprecate any moves to reverse this trend (for example, by using Rampton to relieve overcrowding in other special hospitals) and think that the eventual aim should be to reduce the size of Rampton to 500 or 600 beds. We do not envisage that this would necessarily imply a reduction in staff complement; we think that any potential savings will be largely offset by the additional staff which will be necessary when other of our recommendations are implemented.

5.12   A closed institution

We think that Rampton operates too much as a closed and secretive institution, and that a more open management style should be adopted. Rampton staff have at present to seek prior permission of DHSS before delivering any lecture or publishing any article relating to their official duties. This is unnecessarily restrictive and encourages a closed approach by staff. Any necessary retrictions (eg on confidentiality of personal information about patients or security measures) should be clearly defined and staff should have to do no more than seek the approval of their Head of Department. Heads of Departments and consultants should be left to use their own discretion about consulting the DHSS (or, under the management arrangements we shall be proposing, the Review Board) if controversial issues may arise. Moreover, we think that the staff should be positively encouraged to give factual talks about the hospital to local and professional organisations and to write about their professional work in journals. In the context of this more open management style less emphasis can and should be placed on the provisions of the Official Secrets Act which are in practice unlikely to have to be invoked save in exceptional cases such as those involving the disclosure of the security arrangements at the hospital.

5.13   Patients awaiting discharge and transfer

5.13.1   There are 122 patients in Rampton who in the opinion of all concerned should not be there. These are patients who have been approved for transfer to a NHS hospital, but for whom no place can be found. Over 50 patients, most of them mentally handicapped, have been waiting for over two years. We think this is a scandal. It affects both the welfare of patients—the most important consideration—and the morale of staff, who see all their efforts to prepare patients for life outside Rampton apparently going for nothing. We stress in Chapter 15, where we discuss these issues further, that the responsibility for this state of affairs rests with the NHS, not with Rampton, though we recognise the difficulties under which overcrowded NHS psychiatric (particularly mental handicap) hospitals are working. We think that the recommendations of Mrs Dell's report on the difficulty of transferring patients from Special Hospitals to NHS hospitals should be adopted, and suggest that a joint effort should be made urgently by Rampton and the NHS to find places for mentally handicapped patients who have been on the waiting list for transfer for more than two years. We also recommend that there should be a wider range of programmes for developing patients' independence and self-reliance in preparation for discharge or transfer.

5.13.2   We also think that urgent steps should be taken by the Home Office to speed up their decisions on whether to accept the recommendations of MHRTs to transfer or discharge patients subject to a 'restriction order' (see paragraph 9.1.2(a)). At present, patients have to wait several months after attending a tribunal before a decision can be reached. We find these delays to be intolerable and we do not think that patients should be subjected to the protracted tension and frustration that they cause.

5.14   Management

Finally we believe that Rampton has been bedevilled by a wholly unsatis-factory management structure, one that has tended to make it difficult to get the hospital's problems put right. As we pointed out in paragraph 5.2.1, the structure has in itself obstructed the emergence of the professional leadership whose absence we commented on in that paragraph, and, by confusing executive and consultative functions, has inhibited decision-making at all levels. Our proposals for change in this field (including the appointment of a Medical Director—see paragraph 5.2.3 above) are crucial to the implementation of all our other recommendations, and we think they must be summarised in a separate chapter.

CHAPTER 6

THE MANAGEMENT OF RAMPTON

6.1 Why change is necessary

6.1.1 If the recommendations we are making can be implemented, the result should be to make Rampton a better place for patients and staff. The trouble is that few of our recommendations will be acceptable to everyone, and few therefore will be introduced quickly. Many of them involve the changing of attitudes of staff, and these changes come slowly. Most require a period of consultation with staff interests, because they cannot be imposed from above but require a degree of commitment from staff for their successful implementation.

6.1.2 Rampton in short needs a continuing period of attention beyond that which any Review Team can give. It needs management convinced of the need for change and structured in such a way that, progressively over the next few years, it is able to introduce changes to which staff at all levels are committed.

6.1.3 In our judgement the present management structure is inadequate for its current tasks let alone for taking on the management of the changes which are needed. We have therefore given much thought to the sort of arrangements which will give a good chance of our report and recommendations being implemented. There are two strands to our thinking on this subject. First there is the question of the organisation at official level—the employment of officers to administer the hospital, to manage and guide it in the performance of all its various roles. Secondly there is the question whether a significant change in this official level of management will do all that is needed. Each of these aspects is important and is considered in turn.

6.2 Official management arrangements

6.2.1 Our first proposal, which we summarised in paragraph 5.2.3 above, is that a new post of Medical Director should be created to provide the professional leadership which has been so sadly lacking. A repeated complaint from staff has been the absence of anyone 'in charge' at Rampton. Some staff would clearly be ready to return to the former concept of a Medical Superintendent, a doctor with supreme personal authority to whom all staff and professions are ultimately responsible. As we have already said, we do not favour the return to such an authoritarian and outmoded concept, and we reiterate that we see the Medical Director as leader of a team, with as much emphasis on the team element as the leadership element. He should have some clinical work in order that his job does not become divorced from clinical matters. But his case-load would need to be such as to allow him to devote sufficient time to his management responsibilities.

6.2.2 There should be a Hospital Management Team (HMT) which would consist of the Medical Director as chairman, the Chief Nursing Officer and the Administrator. Its function would be to take day to day decisions affecting the hospital as a whole and to exercise a general oversight of implementation of agreed hospital policy.

6.2.3   The HMT should be assisted by a Heads of Department Committee (HDC). The HDC would be responsible for advising on all across-the-board topics and policy formulation. It would be responsible in particular for drafting the annual operational plan which will provide policy and planning direction to the hospital, and proposals for the allocation of resources amongst the various services at the hospital.

6.2.4   The present Policy Committee should be abolished. It is too large (30 members) and has been an ineffective and unwieldy instrument, which can have no role in our proposed future pattern. The present structure, including the Hospital Executive Committee (the Hospital Administrator, the Chairman of the Consultants Advisory Committee and the Chief Nursing Officer) and the Finance Committee would be superseded by the proposed HMT.

6.2.5   We do not think that the POA or the other staff associations should be represented within the management structure as at present, as this seems to us to confuse management with consultation. Instead we propose that there should be a joint committee of management and representatives of the POA (as the officially recognised body representing Rampton staff), which should meet at regular intervals. Both sides should contribute to the agenda. We think that arrangements of this sort could be devised without difficulty on the basis of the existing formal Whitley Council system.

6.2.6   In addition to good machinery for staff consultation there needs to be an effective system of communication within the hospital if things are to be understood and implemented. We recommend that the hospital should seek the help of a body like the Industrial Society, experienced in instituting effective communication systems.

6.2.7   We spell out these proposals in a little more detail in Chapter 29 where we also deal with the role of the existing multi-disciplinary clinical teams and propose the setting up of a resocialisation team. In the same chapter we also describe in detail the present management structure and the somewhat complicated linkage between the management at local level and the officials of DHSS who play a significant part in the present arrangements.

6.3   A Review Board

6.3.1   The management proposals just described will, we believe, provide a solid foundation for the progressive improvement of conditions for patients and staff in the hospital along the lines we indicate in this report. The HMT will provide professional leadership and take the day to day decisions. The HDC will consider the broad issues which affect all departments with specific responsibilities in regard to advice on policy formulation, the budget and other across-the-board subjects. The pattern we propose is not new and has been well tried elsewhere.

6.3.2   The question we have to ask ourselves is whether these management changes alone will be enough to secure the implementation of the proposals in this report. It is true that superimposed upon our recommended management structure will be the officials of DHSS, able and willing to take a broad view of Rampton's problems based upon the knowledge and experience gained from their responsibilities for the special hospitals as a whole. However the DHSS is remote, and Rampton is but one of the hospitals for which it is directly responsible. It is not easy within a civil service department to ensure continuity of personnel, and as we have said continuing application to Rampton's problems is a prerequisite to progress.

6.3.3   Our recommendations whilst altering the structure, only create one new post, that of Medical Director. The choice of the person to fill this post is clearly crucial, but even assuming the recruitment of an eminently suitable person able to provide dynamic leadership, all the other personnel are likely to be the same. They will be organised in a different and more effective way, and this may release latent initiatives and energy. Nevertheless, we think it is too much to expect that one new appointment and a new structure will do what is needed. Rampton has been reported upon before, and much of what we have to say is not in principle new. It is the implementation of ideas which has proved the stumbling block in the past, and if our efforts are not to be wasted, it is essential to make sound recommendations about implementation. Otherwise our report will, like its predecessors, become one more document for some future committee of inquiry to read.

6.3.4   We consider therefore that for a limited period Rampton needs a new body charged with the specific responsibility of ensuring that the proposals in this report are implemented. We suggest that this body should be called the Rampton Review Board. It would be appointed by and be directly responsible to the Secretary of State to whom it would report regularly. It would be locally based and in regular contact with management and staff at Rampton. We think that the Board should be appointed for a period of three years and that for its period of office should be formally invested with wide supervisory powers, over the running of the hospital, which we describe in Chapter 29. Its existence would ensure that there is a degree of public surveillance of the institution for the next few years. We would expect the Board from the outset to leave the hospital management to get on without interference with the day-to-day administration of the hospital. Towards the end of the three-year period we suggest that the Secretary of State should review the way the Board has operated and consider whether any of its features should be incorporated on a long-term basis in the management arrangements at Rampton or indeed the other special hospitals.

6.3.5   The Board should consist of five or seven members including the Chairman, and we think it is desirable that the majority of them should have local or regional connections so as to ensure that the Board is not seen as a distant and remote body. We think that people with the right experience and qualifications could be found from industry, the universities, the trades unions and the public service, including of course the NHS. We think the Secretary of State should be looking primarily for people with experience of management, in particular the management of change. It would clearly be desirable for some members to have a specific knowledge of hospitals and mental health and to hold appropriate professional qualifications. In order that the thinking and work of the Review Team is available to the Board, some means needs to be found, whether by membership of the Board or otherwise, of associating the Review Team with the Review Board, particularly during the first 12 months of the Board's existence.

6.3.6 The Chairman and members of the Board would all be part-time. Members will however have plenty to do in guiding and supporting the staff at the hospital, and in regularly reviewing its activities by personal visits. We think that the Chairman should be remunerated on the basis of approximately two days' work per week—certainly during the first year after appointment —and members on the basis of half a day per week. The appointments must be of people prepared to spend the time and energy which we believe to be needed.

6.3.7 Under our proposals, there would be no change in the Secretary of State's statutory responsibility for managing the special hospitals, and the staff's existing status as civil servants would remain unchanged. The Secretary of State would continue to be responsible in law and would need to retain such powers as were necessary to ensure uniformity of standard in key areas between one special hospital and another. But subject to this he would delegate to the Board his statutory responsibility for the management of Rampton itself. Means would have to be found of linking the Board to the staff of DHSS concerned with the special hospitals, so that the Review Board can have the benefit of their knowledge and experience.

6.3.8 To sum up, we see the Board in practice as providing an accessible and committed group to whom the HMT can turn for advice and guidance, and who will keep the momentum of change going when those nearer the coal face may be flagging. Although vested with the powers of the Secretary of State (except in regard to reserved matters), we see the Board's main function not primarily as one of giving formal approvals or exercising its authority in a legalistic way, but as supporting, counselling and guiding the Medical Director, the HMT and the HDC. We see the Board as taking part in and guiding the discussions which will be needed with staff interests, and in developing the external relations of the hospital which has for so long been self-contained, inward looking and divorced from the region in which it is set.

6.4 Conclusion

6.4.1 There has been, and we think rightly, considerable public concern about Rampton. There have been criticisms of the regime by former staff members. There have been representations that Rampton should be closed. We doubt whether the public should be satisfied with a report which points the way ahead, but leaves the responsibility for future improvement in the hands of the existing staff, differently organised and supplemented by the appointment of a Medical Director. The appointment of an independent Board of persons of standing, charged with implementing the review proposals, should give the public the confidence that this report will not simply be buried but will be acted upon. We think our proposal for a Board is fully justified to allay public disquiet. The appointment of a Board also gives the promise of real improvement in the future at Rampton, which has been so much reported upon, but where so much remains to be done in spite of the devotion and care which most staff members give to their work.

6.4.2   Patients in particular should be reassured that there is an accessible body to whom they can turn, who although responsible for Rampton have a degree of independence and the powers to deal with any matters which are brought to their attention from any quarter. It is for this reason that in Chapter 30 we have placed squarely upon the shoulders of the Review Board the responsibility for ensuring that the complaints procedure works effectively. Moreover, we draw attention to the fact that of 178 complaints received at Rampton during the period 1974–1978 (see paragraph 30.2.4) not one was substantiated. This fact reinforces our view that the Review Board should give special attention to the way complaints are handled.

ANNEX TO PART I

DAILY LIFE ON THE MALE BLOCK WARDS
(see paragraph 5.3.2)

Note: This Annex was written as a result of observations made in the latter months of 1979 and early months of 1980. Following consultation with management and staff in August 1980, many practices here described have been modified or are being re-examined with a view to change.

Virtually all Rampton patients spend the first two or three years of their stay on a block ward in the high security area of the hospital. Patients on these wards sleep either in single rather cell-like siderooms opening off the main corridor of the ward or in dormitories. Each ward also has a dining room and a day room as well as a kitchen, bedroom, lavatories etc. Bedroom and dormitories contain no furniture except beds, and patients have to keep all personal possessions in lockers in the corridor.

We give below an account of a typical day of a male patient on a block ward. It should be borne in mind however that there are differences between one ward and another, and that there will therefore be various elements in the account below which will not apply to all wards.

1. The day shift arrives

At 7.47 am the day staff arrive on the ward. They assemble in the charge nurses' office, read the reports written since they were last on duty, and note to which area of the ward—dormitory, various corridors, day room etc—they have been allocated. This is the only time of day when the ward team are together as a group; for much of the day, unless they are off the ward escorting patients, they will be stationed in the area of the ward for which they are responsible, observing and supervising patients, avoiding turning their backs on them and keeping in sight and sound of each other as much as possible.

2. The patients get up

As the required minimum staff level to open up each area of the ward is reached, the patients are woken and let out of their rooms. Beds are stripped and searched. Patients who sleep in single rooms put on their slippers (which have been outside their doors during the night) and proceed in single file to the sluice with their chamber pots. (Dormitories all have WCs, so this is not necessary for dormitory patients.)

3. The patients dress

Patients next collect their day clothes from the store. A reliable patient who has earned the job of storeman hands out the clothes. (All 'ward worker' jobs such as storeman are much coveted, because the incumbents earn maximum rewards under the 'points' system.) Each patient has his own number for shoes, clothes, locker key etc. Clothes are taken to the main corridor or the billiard room where patients stand together to dress. Night clothes are then returned to the store.

Patients are expected to wear a tie at all times.

4. Room cleaning

Patients next make their beds and clean the bedrooms or dormitory floor. In some wards floors are swept and buffed with a 'bumper'; in others patients clean the floors on their hands and knees with a floorcloth. When they have finished, patients stand outside their rooms to have them inspected; if they are satisfactory, they are told by the nurse to go and empty their buckets. Rooms and dormitories are then closed to patients for the day.

5. The patients wash

After collecting washing gear, towels and plastic beakers from the lockers patients proceed to the washrooms. With up to 40 residents on some wards queuing is inevitable. On about half the block wards patients shave before breakfast. On those wards where rather more cleaning is done before workshops, shaving is left until the before lunch period. Those patients who prefer not to use electric shavers have to share a small number of safety razors; the blades (which are also communal) can only be removed by the nurses with a special key and are changed daily. In Drake Ward (the high security 'special care unit') patients do not handle razors and are shaved by nursing staff. All of these activities are carried out under close nursing staff supervision. The patients talk little and there is an impression of urgency all the time.

6. Breakfast

While washing and toilet is going on the ward workers are preparing for breakfast. One 'kitchen man' will have brought all the nurses tea as they stand observing the main group of patients dress. Another will have collected the cutlery box from the duty room and laid the tables. Before breakfast patients form a queue in the main corridor and are counted. Breakfast and other meals are served from heated trolleys. It is usual for grace to be said albeit somewhat cursorily. As the patients take their first course at breakfast time, on one ward they show their locker keys to the serving nurse to prove they have not lost them. (On another the toilet gear is actually taken into the dining room.) The most striking aspect of all meal-time in most block wards is that they are invariably silent, although we have not been able to establish whether there is in effect a rule forbidding any talking at all. At breakfast time bread is taken round by a nurse who gives it by hand straight from the bag as each patient requests the number of slices he wants. The seating arrangement is non-institutional, with small tables seating six, each with its own tea pot, although this homely touch is spoilt by the fact that the tea has milk, and on some wards, sugar, added to the pot. The ward workers help serve the other patients with second courses etc, and their own meals are passed out through the kitchen hatch for them to eat later. Second helpings are freely offered, and very little food is wasted. There is a cutlery count before the patients leave the room.

7. After breakfast

Medicines are given after meals; in some wards they are sometimes distributed from a trolley in the dining room, in others patients go in alphabetical order to the duty room or clinic for them. As a precaution against medication being avoided or secreted, water is usually poured on the tablets in the beaker. Lavatories are opened at this time. There is time for a smoke in the free period that follows breakfast but workshop patients soon queue up to change from slippers to shoes and put on their overalls ready to leave soon after 9 am. They form a queue at the end of the corridor and wait for the escort nurse who counts them out. Similarly the education group patients get ready and are checked off the ward. On the admission wards patients going to the Assessment Unit queue up in a separate group.

8. Mornings on the ward

Those remaining on the ward in the mornings are two or three ward workers, newly admitted patients awaiting assessment, sick patients awaiting a visit from the medical officer, patients in seclusion, and all patients on the high security Drake Ward. Apart from those who are sick or in seclusion all patients remaining on the ward work hard. Ward workers make coffee for themselves and the staff once or twice during the morning. Patients on Drake Ward scrub floors and wash down walls throughout the morning. Recently-admitted patients on Cavendish Ward do simple industrial occupational therapy without tools. Once a week at this time the storeman will do all the personal laundry for those patients who have their own clothing, using the ward washing machine.

9. Lunch

When the patients return from workshops etc, between 11.30 am and 11.45 am, they queue for a rub down search before they enter the main corridor of the ward. They then change into their ward slippers, remove their overalls and are free until lunch at 12 mid-day. No one can go to their rooms because sleeping areas are closed; in any case there are no personal possessions there to get at. The routine at lunchtime is similar to that at breakfast.

10. After lunch

After having been given their medicine and used the lavatory, patients who attend the workshops are free until 1 pm and patients who attend the school till 2 pm. They sit in the day/TV room which has chairs in rows and some occasional tables for letter writing or cards. Most nurses sit along the wall of the room watching the TV too, but they are at right angles to the patients and most patients are a yard or two away. If a patient wants to light a cigarette he asks one of the nurses if he can do so; the wall lighter is in the corridor two or three yards from the lounge door. Having lit his cigarette the patient waits on the threshold of the room and says: 'Please can I come in sir?' Staff tend to group together at this time (and during the corresponding period during the evening) reading newspapers, talking to each other or watching TV.

11. Afternoon and early evenings on the ward

At 1 pm, workshop patients go on to the 'airing court' for an hour to play football etc under the supervision of occupations staff. They return to the workshops at 2 pm and at this time or soon after other patients go back to the school for the afternoon session. These activities end at 4.15 pm. Special care ward patients on Drake are 'on court' for an hour during the afternoon and afterwards do simple contract occupational therapy without tools. High tea is at 5 pm and evening classes, which are voluntary, occur between 6.15 and 8.15 pm. There is an evening drink and cake or sausage roll between 7 and 8 pm.

12.   Social and sporting activities

On various evenings of the week block ward patients can attend bingo, films and the weekly social in the main hall or can go swimming or play badminton in the gymnasium. In addition they can watch (but rarely play in) sports matches at the weekends (see paragraph 15).

13.   The patients go to bed

Some patients will go to bed soon after the evening drink, others will stay up until shortly before the night staff come on duty at 9.10 pm. Patients bathe or shower twice a week; there are two baths in each bathroom to enable nurses to supervise a greater number of patients at one time. Final doses of daytime medication are given at bedtime; a very small number of male patients receive night sedation. Patients are then locked into their rooms and dormitories by the day staff. They are allowed to keep their lights on to enable them to read for an hour or two.

14.   Night routine

There is one night nurse per ward; communicating doors between the block wards are kept open to permit contact between nurses. Night nurses can observe patients through small holes in the doors of side rooms or through the glass doors of the dormitories. Patients requiring nursing or medical attention having attracted a nurse's attention need to wait until a second staff member has been called before their door can be opened at night. Night charge nurses and relief staff nurses have hand radio sets to enable them to provide assistance quickly in an emergency.

15.   Weekends

The routine described above is modified at weekends when patients do not attend school or workshops. There is extra cleaning on Saturday mornings—polish is applied then to many of the floors. There is visiting on Saturday and Sunday afternoons, and block ward patients are allowed to watch sports matches on Sunday morning. Patients can attend services in the hospital chapel on Sunday.

PART II

CHAPTER 7

THE 'RAMPTON SYSTEM'

7.1 The 'System' described

7.1.1 The range of treatment which Rampton patients have the right to expect should be broadly comparable to that available in NHS mental illness and mental handicap hospitals and should be limited only by security considerations. Rampton does in theory offer a wide range of treatments—individual psychotherapy, chemotherapy, behaviour modification programmes, specific social training, remedial education and workshop training. However, some of these specific treatment methods and therapies play only a relatively small part in total care compared with the process which we have come to think of and describe as the 'Rampton system'. This is a regime to which every patient is subjected and consists of an elaborate system of incentives and disincentives built into every aspect of a patient's life by which he or she is 'encouraged' to conform to the norms of behaviour which Rampton considers to be appropriate.

7.1.2 The application of the principles within this regime are demonstrated in the way patients progress or otherwise through the hospital. This follows a standard pattern from which deviations appear to be rare. (We understand that some statistical research is being carried out at the hospital with a view to demonstrating how common such deviations in fact are. An unrestricted patient can, of course, be discharged by the MHRT at any stage in his Rampton career.) An average of six months for both male and female patients is spent on the respective admission wards. In this period patients are assessed by various methods within the Assessment Unit (see paragraph 9.3). From the admission ward they move to one of the block wards (situated, as is the admission ward, in the central high security area of the hospital), where on the male side conditions are very austere (see Chapter 11). If patients 'progress', in the sense that if their degree of conformity is considered satisfactory by the staff, many of them can expect to spend between two and three years on a block ward. From there the significant move is made to a villa ward in the less secure outer area of the hospital, with a notably higher standard of comfort, amenities and privileges (see Chapter 14). There are three main categories of villa, preliminary, preparatory and pre-discharge, with a progressively higher standard of amenity; the principle is, though this is not always practicable or necessary, that the patient will spend a period in a villa of each category. After a period in the villas the majority of patients, again given satisfactory progress, can be expected to be transferred to NHS hospitals or discharged (see Chapter 15). Any patient who has episodic or prolonged periods of disturbed behaviour may require removal for varying periods to a special care block ward where there is an enhanced staff/patient ratio and greater emphasis both on security and on the application of a rigid routine which we describe in paragraph 13.3.

7.1.3 It is reasonable that different patients should be treated in different environments to reflect their differing therapeutic needs. Moreover as a patient responds to treatment it is only to be expected that he will require less supervision and can be treated in less austere and functional surroundings. At Rampton, however, the various degrees of amenity and privilege characteristic of different parts of the hospital are themselves used as incentives and disincentives to encourage patients to modify their behaviour. Patients are offered the prospect of progressing as quickly as possible to a more attractive environment if their behaviour 'improves', and threatened with the possibility of moving back into a less attractive one if it deteriorates.

7.2   The advantages and disadvantages of the 'system'

7.2.1   We want to stress at this stage that we do not think it is wrong in principle to use rather simple 'reformatory' techniques such as those described above on the sort of patients to be found in Rampton. Those techniques were widely used in mental handicap hospitals 30 years ago and, for some patients they may still, in the present state of knowledge, be the best form of 'treatment' available. We also want to stress that in our view the majority of the staff at Rampton are doing their best, often under extremely difficult circumstances, to operate the system as fairly and humanely as they can. Nevertheless, there are clearly inherent dangers and potential problems in operating policies of this sort, to all of which we think Rampton has to a degree succumbed.

7.2.2   First, there is the danger of inflexibility, that all or most categories of patient will be subject to the same routine, irrespective of individual needs. Secondly, a disciplined heavily-structured framework of care, with the emphasis on compliance with (mostly unwritten) rules, will accustom patients to rely on external rather than internal sources of control and inhibit the development of self-awareness, self-reliance and self-control. Thirdly, staff may be tempted to adopt inappropriate criteria for deciding patients' progress through the system, or awarding or withholding privileges generally and use their own imposed and artificial standards of 'good behaviour'. Finally, there is a risk that because the requirements of security place a limit on the incentives which can be offered, the disincentives will be correspondingly overdone and at the 'bottom end' of the system an unacceptably harsh regime and an unreasonably low threshold of personal comfort and amenity will be imposed.

7.2.3   The rest of this chapter is largely concerned with the first three of the pitfalls listed above; the fourth chiefly arises in the context of the regime on the male block wards, which we discuss in Chapter 11.

7.2.4   We should mention in this context that since 1975 Rampton has had an Ethics Committee whose purpose has been defined as being to safeguard patients' human rights in so far as these may be affected by their treatment and management, and to provide a source of reference or guidance within the hospital for staff involved in treatment or research programmes. It does not appear to us that this Committee has been as active as it might have been in monitoring some of the potential dangers of the 'system' and we suggest that its future role in this area might profitably be reviewed.

7.3   Towards a more flexible system

7.3.1   One important aspect of the inflexibility of the present 'system' is that although there are a few wards which specialise in either mental handicap or mental illness most wards at Rampton accommodate a mix of patients with a wide range of mental disorders and clinical needs, all of whom are subjected to the same ward regime whether or not it is appropriate to them personally. Whilst it can be argued that some degree of mix or dispersal of certain kinds of clinical problem can be helpful, we think this is generally true only where small numbers are involved. Where the range of intelligence and kinds of disability are wide, the general policy and regime of the ward can be suitable only for a limited number of patients. Attempts are being made at the hospital to achieve a better streaming or 'peer-grouping' arrangement on more wards. We support these attempts, and think they should be pursued more energetically.

7.3.2   Even more important is the need for a wider range of individual treatment programmes for patients, on whatever ward they may be. Theoretically the individual needs of each patient, based on multidisciplinary observation and assessment, are taken into account in planning therapeutic, occupational, rehabilitative and educational programmes. In practice however it often seems more a question of fitting the patient into the system than of devising ways to suit the patient's needs. We recognise, of course, that in any large hospital it will always be difficult to strike the proper balance between the needs of individuals and those of patients in general, but we do not believe that the undoubted need for orderly routines on the wards should preclude each patient having a properly designed individual treatment programme.

7.3.3   We have observed that consultants' direct involvement with the care of individual patients is frequently limited, apart from at case conferences (see paragraph 7.4.2 below) and when submissions have to be prepared for MHRTs. A part-time consultant psychotherapist has recently been appointed; we think this is a step in the right direction, and that individual psychotherapy and discussion groups should be encouraged. It seems likely that many patients would benefit from behaviour modification, self-care and social skills programmes, including ward-based programmes run mainly by nursing staff; at present very little can be offered in this area, largely because of the recent acute shortage at Rampton of clinical psychologists, and, to a lesser extent, social workers. We think it is essential that urgent steps should be taken to increase the clinical psychology involvement in treatment programmes at Rampton; we make specific recommendations in Chapter 25 for increasing the number of clinical psychologists working at Rampton. There might also be a need for additional nursing staff in some areas to operate the sort of programmes we have in mind.

7.3.4   The third aspect of the inflexibility of the 'system' to which we wish to draw particular attention is the segregation of male and female patients and staff. This segregation is universal on the wards and in most of the occupations department. There is however a limited amount of integration in some other areas. The Assessment Unit (see paragraph 9.3) is mixed, although patients return to their segregated wards for meals and at nights. We found it paradoxical that the only time during their time at Rampton that patients were able to mix freely during the day with other patients and staff of the opposite sex was when they had just been admitted and the staff had as yet had no first-hand knowledge of any dangerous sexual or other tendencies. In the occupations department only the print shop and the garden working party are integrated. Classes in the patients' education department are mixed, as are the playgroups and other activities for the severely handicapped run by the nurses of the Activity Group (see Chapter 21). There are also some closely supervised mixed social activities in the evening, such as the weekly socials, bingo sessions and film shows.

7.3.5   Integration of the sexes is an emotive subject amongst Rampton staff and this is hardly surprising, particularly in the light of the fact that many of Rampton's male patients have a history of sexual offences, often associated with marked social inadequacies. We fully understand the misgivings which some Rampton staff have expressed at the prospect of further integration, and it would be unrealistic to claim that any moves in this direction might not involve some additional risks both to other patients and to staff. However, we saw examples of such integration working successfully in institutions in Holland. Moreover the potential value of integration as a contribution towards realistic resocialisation programmes for patients of both sexes is so great that in our view some careful further extension would in any case be justified; we think that some of the workshops might be good places to start (see paragraph 23.4.3).

7.3.6   Finally, we think that the present security regime is imposed too uniformly in all areas of the hospital, and that there is scope in this area for more flexibility. We elaborate further on this in paragraph 8.6.

7.3.7   If the recommendations in paragraphs 7.3.1–7.3.6 were adopted, we think that this would in itself go a long way towards meeting the second of the pitfalls inherent in the Rampton system which we listed in paragraph 7.3.2, the over-emphasis on rules and external controls. A more flexible 'patient centred' approach, with less emphasis on compliance with rules for their own sake, ought to provide more opportunities for patients to express themselves, to co-operate responsibly in their treatment and rehabilitation, to exercise more choice, and to be more involved in decision-taking. We believe that substantial moves could be made in this direction without any significant reduction in levels of security. There would certainly be staffing and other implications to be considered.

7.4   How patients' progress through the system is determined

7.4.1   All patients in Rampton are compulsorily detained under the Mental Health Act, and under the provisions of the Act (or, in the case of 'restricted' patients, as a matter of administrative practice) their legal status is subject to formal review at regular intervals—see paragraph 15.5.3. But, as a wholly separate exercise, patients' cases are also reviewed from time to time to determine their progress through the 'system' and their suitability for education, workshop training or other therapeutic or rehabilitational procedures. Case conferences are the main method used to carry out such reviews.

7.4.2   Case conferences are quite formal affairs, and can involve up to a dozen members of staff as well as the patient. The consultant in charge of the patient's case takes the chair; the other people normally present are the charge nurse and nursing officer responsible for the patient's current ward, the charge nurses of any wards to which he might possibly be transferred, the medical assistant who is normally involved in his care and representatives of the education, occupations, social work and (where this is possible in the light of current staffing problems) clinical psychology departments. The staff usually discuss the case among themselves, and the patient (wearing his 'Sunday best') is then called in to answer questions and give his own views. If sensitively chaired, case conferences on these lines can provide a useful forum for multidisciplinary discussion of patients' progress and needs. Some conferences which we attended however were too formally run, with no real discussion of options, and were in consequence in our view less useful than they could have been; we were not surprised to be told that many patients find them stressful occasions. We think that there should be a review of the way case conferences are run. This could include consideration of the possibility of relatives in some cases being present for part of the conferences, although we recognise that there are real problems in such a proposal.

7.4.3. The frequency of case conferences is not prescribed by law or regulation and is a matter for the consultant in charge. In practice all patients have an initial 'planning' case conference after they have been assessed (see paragraph 9.4). As a minimum there is then another conference before a patient is moved to a villa, and a final one before discharge or transfer. In addition there are other reviews from time to time. We think that patients' progress should be subject to formal review at least annually, and this will be easier to achieve if the total population at Rampton can be further reduced. But we think that an improved clinical information system for consultants would meanwhile enable a better track to be kept of patients' progress, as well as providing information about any delays and bottlenecks in the system.

7.4.4 Much emphasis is placed at case conferences on the patient's behaviour and whether or not he or she has conformed with the high or artificial norms of behaviour which are expected under the nursing regime on the block wards. Little account may often be taken of relevant dynamic social or other factors. Moreover in the case of patients who have been convicted in the courts it appears that the nursing staff, who in practice often dominate case conferences and have the major say in determining patients' progress through the 'system', will often relate the time a patient should spend on a block ward, or in Rampton, to the severity of the original offence as much as to his current clinical needs. We think that there should be wide discussion within the hospital on the criteria used for determining progress through the 'system', and that in the light of these discussions more explicit guidelines should be promulgated.

CHAPTER 8

SECURITY

8.1 We do not think it is helpful to express a view as to which of the two functions of a special hospital—security and treatment—should be considered the more important. Both are important and the way the hospital is run must clearly reflect both functions adequately. This is easily said, but, as we pointed out in paragraph 2.2.5, the interests of security and those of treatment sometimes conflict. Compromises, inevitably imperfect in that they can wholly satisfy neither interest, will very often be required. Well-meaning outside observers of Rampton may sometimes we think, tend to underplay the importance of security. It is easy to forget that a patient whose behaviour in the controlled and structured environment of Rampton seems normal and innocuous enough may have committed terrible offences before his admission. In spite of the treatment he has received there may be uncertainty as to whether he will commit offences again if he is able to abscond before he has been judged ready for discharge. On the other hand the staff at Rampton may sometimes be tempted to seek to give security priority over virtually all other considerations. This attitude is understandable. In the first place staff (and their families living near the hospital) may see themselves as particularly at risk in the event of any breach of security. Secondly, any escapes tend to be blamed upon staff and if the escape is followed by violence or crime, the public are naturally critical of the security arrangements. To give security absolute priority is nevertheless an attitude which we cannot endorse. Anything approaching total security would only be achieved at the expense of most if not all therapeutic activity, and this would be unacceptable. But the fact must be faced that any relaxation in security will have some additional risk of harm to staff, other patients and people outside the hospital; the decision as to whether in any particular case the extra risk is worth taking in the light of the therapeutic or other benefits which can be obtained in return is certainly -amongst the most difficult and sensitive ones which those responsible for patient care at Rampton have to take. They deserve all the help and support they can get in arriving at their decision, and we think it is right that decisions should normally be taken only after full interdisciplinary discussion (see paragraph 15.5.2).

8.2 The public at large probably place the greatest importance upon the security aspect of a special hospital and some people would be content to see mentally ill offenders locked away for very long periods. Nevertheless those who work with the mentally ill person of dangerous or criminal tendencies must not see their role in too simple terms. It is much more than a security exercise and its challenge is to reconcile the need for treatment with the requirements of security.

8.3 The Chief Nursing Officer has overall responsibility for security at Rampton; a Security Adviser, who is a nursing officer, reports to him. Day to day security is largely in practice the responsibility of the nursing staff. We have considered whether we should recommend a separate security staff at Rampton, leaving the nursing staff responsible for purely nursing duties. We found a pattern of this sort in some of the institutions we visited in Holland. We think however that the disadvantages of introducing any such system at Rampton would outweigh any possible advantages. The additional staff cost would be substantial. More importantly, if one group of Rampton staff were given specific and exclusive responsibility for security, everyone else would tend to become very much less security conscious and the standard of security throughout the hospital as a whole would be likely to fall seriously. We do not therefore recommend any changes on these lines.

8.4   Our general views on the practical aspects of security can be summarised as follows. Firstly, we think that the existing security systems at Rampton are by and large good ones which are operated effectively. We make some detailed suggestions for minor improvements in the next section of this chapter; none of them should have any noticeable impact on patients' daily life or interfere in any way with therapeutic programmes. Secondly, we think there may be a tendency for staff to rely uncritically on security considerations in deciding against improvements which could be introduced in patients' quality of life or treatment regimes; we give some examples of this in Chapter 11. We think that when proposals for such improvements are being considered a careful and realistic assessment of the security risks involved should always be made, and that it should be accepted by all concerned that a certain amount of security risk may have to be tolerated for the sake of the treatment or other benefits which can be gained in return. Finally, we think that there is scope for a more flexible approach to security in the villa areas and that the present practice of applying uniformly high standards of security to virtually every part of the hospital could be modified. We elaborate on this in section 8.6 of this chapter.

8.5   The operation of existing security systems

8.5.1   The standard of security attained at Rampton may be judged by its record, in that during the last ten years there has been only a total of 17 escape incidents of which eight have occurred from outside working parties, five from villas or visiting rooms and four from within the high security area. In most of these incidents the absconders have been returned very soon, from within a short distance of the hospital, either by the staff or by the police. Despite this creditable record it is the case that in some areas where high security is essential there are current practices which are not in keeping with the requirements of good security working. There are also deficiencies in materials and resources which could well hinder the attainment and maintenance of satisfactory standards.

8.5.2   The questionable practices within the high security area are mainly concerned with the safety of keys and their usage. We noticed that some senior staff do not carry their security keys upon the leather belt and thong issued for this purpose. It is a common practice to leave security doors open to be locked by members of staff 'following on' behind the staff member who initially opens the door. Security keys are often taken outside the secure area, on outside working parties, to the staff dining rooms and, we were informed, on occasions to staff's homes during meal times. These practices create unnecessary risks and are not acceptable in the maintenance of good security where the basic and elementary principles must always be the security of keys and the elimination of opportunities by which keys may be compromised. We recommend that local management should give urgent consideration to eliminating these practices.

8.5.3 The deficiencies in materials and resources are mainly concerned with the arrangements for emergency security communications and the provision of a satisfactory control room. In the past the UHF radios in general use at the hospital have, due to their age and worn condition, not given satisfactory service; this unacceptable state of affairs has however recently been satisfactorily resolved by the issue of new equipment. Similarly the control room had, at the time of our visits to the hospital, many unsatisfactory aspects. It was physically insecure, the system for issuing and recording security keys was not satisfactory, the storage of reserve keys was not secure and not all staff had been given the benefit of professional training in control room duties. All these deficiencies are now, we understand, being rectified. A new site has been agreed for a control room in which the key-room facilities will operate more efficiently with the incorporation of a key shute and the use of a 'tally' system. It has been agreed that the telephone, UHF, fire alarms display boards and any future alarm systems that may be incorporated will terminate in the control room. Reserve security keys are now stored in a special safe in the charge of the Security Adviser. We think it is essential that adequate training should be provided for controllers, watchkeepers and operators. We understand that courses are now being arranged at HM Prison Staff College for all control room staff.

8.5.4 We recommend that security, fire precautions and health and safety at work should be treated as separate parts of the curriculum in the School of Nursing, rather than merely being included as aspects of general nurse training as at present. Regular one-day refresher training courses should also be held for all staff.

8.6 A more flexible approach to security

8.6.1 There is already differentiation in the level of perimeter security between the outer villa ward area, which is surrounded by a medium security sunken wall and ditch with a 17 foot high chain link fence, and the inner block wards, which are enclosed within an 18 foot concrete wall as well. But physical security within the villa area is the same as that on the block wards. All patients are locked into their bedrooms or dormitories at night, and villa patients must all be escorted wherever they go within the medium secure area; there is no 'ground parole' as at other special hospitals. This applies even to the patients in the male pre-release villas, Sweet Briar and Moss Rose, which are outside the outer perimeter fence altogether and are protected only by their own garden fences. We think it is undesirable that the same strict rules are applied to all patients the day before discharge as are applied to those newly admitted.

8.6.2 In our view, there are many patients in the villa wards at Rampton to whom a high security regime of the kind described is inappropriate. First and foremost there are the 122 patients who have already been approved

41

for discharge or transfer from Rampton, but for whom a place in a NHS hospital or sheltered accommodation has not yet been found. We discuss in Chapter 15 the problems of getting patients discharged or transferred from Rampton; NHS hospitals may be reluctant to accept Rampton patients because of the fact that nothing recent can be known of their behaviour in medium or low security conditions. Secondly, the undifferentiated security regime restricts the opportunities for testing suitable patients in a relaxed environment to see whether they are yet ready to be considered for discharge or transfer. Finally, we think there are probably a substantial number of patients in Rampton who, although not at present approved for discharge or transfer or likely to be so in the near future, do not need to be treated in conditions of very high security, the sort of patients who would be suitable for transfer to medium security units in NHS hospitals if more such units existed.

8.6.3   We think it is wrong in principle to subject patients to a higher degree of security than is clinically necessary, and that if a less rigorous regime could be developed in selected areas of the hospital, a more demanding, encouraging and stimulating life could be provided for many patients with greater opportunities for realistic resocialisation programmes and a much more challenging and fulfilling role for the nursing staff.

8.6.4   We recommend therefore that an immediate study should be put in hand of possible ways of introducing a less rigorous security regime in some villa wards. We recognise that the present lay-out of the hospital does not lend itself to a fully fledged system of 'ground parole', although there may be scope for some moves in this direction.

CHAPTER 9

SELECTION, ADMISSION AND ASSESSMENT

9.1 How patients are selected

9.1.1 Special hospitals are institutions for persons subject to detention under the Mental Health Act who in the Secretary of State's opinion require treatment under conditions of special security on account of their dangerous, violent or criminal propensities. Selection of patients for Rampton and the other special hospitals is thus placed firmly in the hands of the Secretary of State, and therefore, in practice, of the DHSS.

9.1.2 Applications for special hospital places come to DHSS from three main sources:—

a. Prisons or remand centres, in respect of people who have been charged with an offence and are awaiting a court appearance. If a court is satisfied (on the evidence of two medical practitioners) that an offender is suffering from a mental disorder such as to warrant detention in hospital (not necessarily a special hospital), and provided a hospital bed can be made available within 28 days, it can subject to certain restrictions make an order (under Section 60 of the Mental Health Act) that he should be detained in hospital on approximately the same conditions as a 'civil' patient subject to compulsory detention under the Act. If it thinks it necessary for the protection of the public, the Court can also add a 'restriction order' (under Section 65 of the Mental Health Act) which means that the offender cannot be transferred, granted leave, or discharged from hospital without the consent of the Home Secretary. If the referring doctor (usually the Prison Medical Officer considers that the patient, if found guilty of the offence with which he has been charged, should be detained in a *special* hospital on account of his 'dangerous, violent or criminal propensities', he will in advance of the trial ask DHSS for a provisional place pending the outcome of the trial.

b. NHS psychiatric hospitals in respect of non-offender patients who are usually already compulsorily detained under the provisions of the Mental Health Act and whose behaviour is such that special security is required. The referring doctor is usually the consultant psychiatrist in charge of the case.

c. The Home Office, in respect of prisoners who are suffering from a mental disorder. They can be transferred to hospital by an order under Sections 72 or 73 of the Mental Health Act and can be admitted to a special hospital if they require treatment under conditions of special security.

9.1.3 In addition, every year there is a small number of patients referred to DHSS by the Home Office under the provisions of the Criminal Procedure (Insanity) Act 1964. These are persons charged with an offence who have been found 'not guilty by reason of insanity' (under the 'M'Naghten Rules') or 'under disability in relation to trial' (what used to be called 'unfit to plead'), and who need to be detained under conditions of special security. There are

43

special difficulties about the detention of people as a result of alleged offences when their guilt has never been established. These difficulties were recognised by the Butler Committee* on mentally abnormal offenders, who made some recommendations in this area. We understand these recommendations are still under consideration by the Government.

9.1.4 Before sending details of the case to DHSS, the referring doctor will sometimes seek the opinion of a special hospital consultant on the suitability or otherwise of the patient for admission to a special hospital. At present this seems to involve consultants from Broadmoor more often than those from Rampton. Whilst we recognise that DHSS must have the final say on admissions (in view of the Government's ultimate responsibility for law and order and the safety of the public recognised in the statutory provisions about admissions) we think that referring doctors should be actively encouraged to seek the views of Rampton consultants on potential admissions before making formal application to DHSS. The experienced opinion of the Rampton consultants will always be valuable in reducing the number of unsuitable applications. Involving them more in the selection process will add further interest and stimulus to their work as well as reducing their professional isolation. It might also in some instances facilitate the eventual transfer of the patient back into the NHS—see paragraph 15.6.8.

9.1.5 At the DHSS, applications for admission to special hospitals are normally considered by an informal office committee consisting of administrators and a psychiatrist. It has first to be decided whether the patient is suitable for admission to a special hospital and then, if so, which one. DHSS have told us that in deciding the question of suitability for special hospital care, the matters they take into account are whether the patient is properly liable to detention under the Mental Health Act (which includes, in the case of people suffering from psychopathic disorder, an opinion as to whether the disorder requires or is likely to respond to hospital treatment); and whether the patient's 'dangerous, violent or criminal propensities' are such as to require treatment under conditions of special security. In considering the latter question, they tell us that they find the Butler Committee's definition of 'dangerousness' a helpful one, ie 'a propensity to cause serious physical injury or lasting psychological harm'.

9.1.6 As pointed out in paragraph 2.4.6, one of the reasons that the size and nature of the patient population in the special hospitals has substantially changed in recent years appears to be changes in the way that DHSS have interpreted and applied the criteria for admission. We think it important that DHSS should ensure that referring agencies are informed of the way in which the statutory criteria are applied and also that they should carefully monitor continuing trends both in total referrals and in acceptances as essential for effective future planning.

9.1.7 There is one aspect of the admission criteria for special hospitals particularly affecting Rampton on which we think we should comment. We think it inappropriate, other than in exceptional circumstances, for *severely*

---

*Report of the Committee on Mentally Abnormal Offenders. Cmnd 6244. HMSO October 1975.

mentally handicapped patients to be treated in special hospitals. We recognise that the number of severely handicapped patients whose management problems are such that they require the level of security which only a special hospital can provide is very small indeed, and that far fewer such patients are nowadays admitted to special hospitals (eight or nine a year now compared with about 40 a year ten years ago). Nevertheless we think the DHSS should clearly indicate to those concerned that applications for special hospital care for severely mentally handicapped patients will not normally be accepted.

9.1.8 When it has been decided that a patient is suitable for special hospital care, he or she is allocated to a particular hospital. As we explained in paragraph 2.1.4, virtually all mentally handicapped patients and most of the less intelligent of the mentally ill and of those suffering from psychopathic disorder go either to Rampton or to Moss Side (depending on where their home is, what the vacancy position is at each hospital, and, to some extent, their age—younger patients tend to go to Moss Side). Most of the more intelligent mentally ill and psychopathic patients go to Broadmoor or Park Lane, though some may be sent to Rampton where there are usually more vacancies.

9.1.9 When the decision is taken that a patient should be admitted to Rampton, the hospital is notified and all relevant information sent to the Administrator's Department. The hospital then makes arrangements for admission; latterly it has sometimes not been possible to arrange this immediately, if there is pressure on the admission wards. If the patient has been seen before admission by a Rampton consultant, that consultant will usually be responsible for his care in the hospital; otherwise he will be allocated to a consultant on a rota basis.

9.2 The admission wards

9.2.1 All male patients are admitted to Cavendish Ward and all females to Elizabeth Ward. Cavendish has 22 beds and Elizabeth 18, all in single rooms. Elizabeth Ward has a dual function: as well as taking new female admissions it also takes from all the female block wards the physically ill patients who require a high level of nursing care. The needs of these two groups are clearly very different, and this can create nursing difficulties. Moreover neither group of patients has a particularly beneficial effect on the other, and we think the possibility of providing alternative facilities for the physically ill should be examined.

9.2.2 The regimes on the admission wards, both male and female, are typical of those in the other block wards, which we describe in detail in Chapters 11 and 12. The fact however that all six consultants on the male side have patients on Cavendish and both consultants on the female side have patients in Elizabeth makes it more difficult than it would otherwise be to ensure consistent and positive ward policies. We think there would be strong advantages in all patients on the admission wards being under the care of one consultant or at least one consultant being specifically nominated as having particular responsibility for ward policies.

9.2.3　Virtually all patients spend four to six months on the admission wards. (Readmissions tend to move on faster than new admissions as a truncated assessment programme is often possible.) But only eight to twelve weeks is usually spent on actual assessment procedures in the Assessment Unit (see next paragraph). Patients spend an average of nine weeks on the wards before formal assessment starts: and there is usually a delay of some weeks between the completion of assessment and the initial 'planning' case conference which decide where the patient is to move to. We suggest in the next section that there could be more flexibility as to the length of the assessment procedures; we also think it is important that patients should not have to spend longer than is absolutely necessary waiting for assessment or for their planning case conference (although we recognise that in the case of patients who are seriously disturbed on admission time must be allowed for their behaviour to stabilise). We think the improved clinical information system for consultants which we recommend earlier (paragraph 7.4.3) might be helpful in identifying and dealing with bottlenecks in this area.

9.3　The Assessment Unit

9.3.1　The Assessment Unit for both male and female patients is housed in a converted block ward in the inner secure area. Up to 20 patients attend each day and return to the male or female admission wards for meals and at nights. The unit is staffed by a charge nurse (together with two learners from the nurse training school), two occupations officers and two female escorts who attend with the female patients. The observation and assessment procedure covers the clinical signs and symptoms, behaviour problems, manual dexterity and aptitudes, social competence and interaction and educational attainments covering basic discrimination of colour, size, number and time. Each patient's behaviour is recorded daily by the assessment team. At the end of the assessment period, a summary report is produced by the charge nurse highlighting areas of need such as social incompetence, educational deficiencies and so on, which are presented at the planning case conference.

9.3.2　Exceptionally, the assessment period may last as little as six weeks, but eight to twelve weeks is the norm. Our impression is that a substantial number of patients may not need such a prolonged period of assessment, and we think that the possibility of introducing more flexibility into the system should be investigated.

9.3.3　We are concerned that staffing difficulties in the clinical psychology department have meant that the psychology input into the work of the Assessment Unit has been obviously reduced. We regard this as a vital area for clinical psychology involvement, and stress again the urgent need to recruit more professionals in this field—see Chapter 25.

9.3.4　The Assessment Unit sometimes has problems because relief staff are not available to cover either for the charge nurse or for the occupations staff during periods of leave or sickness. We think it desirable that staff should be trained for this purpose. We also suggest that the Unit should be used as a training experience for newly appointed occupations staff and included in induction courses.

9.4 After assessment

A few weeks after the formal assessment period is completed, the initial 'planning' case conference is held, where decisions are taken as to the ward to which the patient will move, and his education and training programme. Occasionally male severely mentally handicapped patients will move straight to Hollies Villa at this stage, but most patients will automatically be transferred to a block ward first. We describe the regime on these wards in more detail in Chapter 11 and 12.

CHAPTER 10

THE ORGANISATION OF THE PATIENT'S DAY

10.1   At this stage in our report, we think we should explain how the daily timetable of every Rampton patient, whether in a block ward or villa, is organised, why we think this timetable is unsatisfactory, and how we think changes could be made. We must start by briefly describing the current nursing shift system (at charge nurse level and below), as it is this which to a very large extent determines the general shape of the patient's daily timetable.

10.2   Rampton operates what is generally known as the 'long day' shift system. There are only two changes of shift in each 24 hour period. The day shift comes on duty at 7.47 am and stays on until 9.30 pm (with 45 minutes lunch break and 40 minutes tea break). The night shift come on duty at 9.10 pm and goes off at 8.04 am. Generally speaking, a nurse on the day shift works only alternate days. There are thus in effect two complete day staffs at Rampton, each working alternate days and not as a normal rule coming into contact with each other. Liaison between shifts is part of the unit nursing officers' responsibility. These officers work two days on duty and two days off to overlap with both shifts of ward staff.

10.3   The shift system means that day staff have to have both their lunch and their tea within their working day. Lunch and tea breaks are taken in three relays based on grade, with the most junior staff going first and the most senior last—the so-called 'three messes'—with the effect that there is a period of two and a quarter hours at lunchtime and two hours at teatime—times when the maximum number of patients are present on the wards—when wards are not fully manned.

10.4   The effect of these arrangements on the patients' daily timetable can be summarised as follows:

a.   The patient's day cannot begin until the day staff are on duty and must end before the night staff come on duty. Patients thus have an unduly long time in bed and a correspondingly short time up. This has many undesirable results. To enable patients to get to work or school by a reasonable hour in the morning they have to get up, wash, have breakfast and receive medication in the space of an hour. The urgency means they have little privacy in the bathrooms and washrooms, and leaves no time for any training in self-help skills. It also often results in frustration-induced aggression. At the other end of the day, the early bedtime seriously curtails evening activities.

b.   Because staff mealtimes have to be spread over such a long period and patients can only be escorted to and from the school when the wards are fully manned, the working day for those attending the school is kept unduly short.

10.5   The patients' daily timetable is as follows (see also the Annex to

48

Part I). Patients are got up as soon as possible after the day staff come on duty, normally between 7.50 am and 8.00 am. There is a ruling that patients cannot be released from their rooms in the morning until there is a full complement of day staff on duty; as a consequence of sickness or absence, there may have to be a reallocation of staff, further delaying the opening of rooms. Having washed and, on the male and some female block wards, cleaned their rooms, patients have breakfast at about 8.15 am. There is usually some ward cleaning done immediately after breakfast. Patients for the work-shops are collected from the wards by occupations staff soon after 9.00 am; patients for the education department have to be escorted there by nurses—teachers are not allowed to escort patients—and it is usually 9.30 am and occasionally as late as 10.00 am before they arrive at the education department. Patients have to be back on the wards for lunch, which is from 12.00 to 1.00 pm. Between 1.00 pm and 2.00 pm workshop patients have an exercise period, weather permitting, on the so-called 'airingcourts' under the supervision of occupations staff, and return to the workshops at 2.00 pm. Patients going to the education department however have to stay on the ward until nurses can be spared to escort them, but as this is dependent on the last of the ward nursing staff returning from lunch, it is often 2.30 pm or later before they get back to their classes. All patients have to be back on the wards for high tea at 5.00 pm (so all three main meals meals are taken within a nine hour period). Evening classes and social activities take place between 6.15 and 8.15 pm. By 8.30 pm all patients are back on their wards and as a general rule, with some exceptions on the female villas, locked into their rooms or dormitories by 9.00 pm, ten minutes before the night shift come on duty. Patients in single rooms are allowed to read or, in the case of villa patients, listen to the radio in bed for an hour or so, before going to sleep.

10.6   We believe that the timetable outlined above is unsatisfactory. Whilst we accept that hospital life must always work to a somewhat different routine from that in the outside world, we think that the routine at Rampton so distorts most people's normal daily life patterns that it must quite seriously jeopardise the hospital's efforts to prepare patients for life in the outside world. We think it is particularly unreasonable that patients should have to be locked in their bedrooms for about 11 hours every night. What may have once had some justification as a routine for severely mentally handicapped patients seems to us increasingly inappropriate for the differing kind of patients who now predominate at Rampton. No doubt some patients will have 'had enough' by 8.30 in the evening, and be ready for a bit of peace and quiet in their room or dormitory. But we cannot believe that this is true of the majority of patients who we are sure would benefit from more extended evening activities, even if this were just informal mixing with other patients and staff.

10.7   We cannot avoid the conclusion that the key to improvements in the patients' daily timetable is to make changes in the nurses' shift system. We recognise of course that this is a controversial area. It was an attempt to implement the recommendations on changing the shift system which the HAS had made in 1971 which led to industrial action at Rampton in 1972 and the subsqent investigation by Mr James Elliott. Mr Elliott himself suggested that the staff should be invited to bring forward proposals for trial work schedules

49

which were not subject to the objections levelled against the present system, and that these schedules should be operated on an experimental basis in a designated ward or unit by those staff who were prepared to do so. But, the Department told us, it was decided that evaluation of alternative shift systems should not be attempted 'until the general climate at the hospital had improved as a result of other changes'. No further action on the shift system has in fact been taken.

10.8   We do not offer any definite blueprint for the changes in the shift system which will be necessary to meet the objections to the present system which we have outlined. We think that Mr Elliott's suggestion, that detailed proposals should come from the staff themselves, was a good one, and we think a similar approach should be adopted now. We recognise that any radical changes could involve some quite considerable disruption of staff's own life patterns and domestic arrangements, particularly where husband and wife are working on alternate days or where nurses have taken a second job on their days off. Any proposals for change would clearly have to take account of these factors. But we are convinced that change must happen, and that further delay in tackling a problem which was first indentified nearly ten years ago would be indefensible.

10.9   Finally, we should make it clear that although we think the main objection to the present shift system is its effect on the patients' daily timetable, we recognise that it has other very serious drawbacks as well. As Mr Elliott recognised, the 'long day' might mean that many staff will become too tired in the last four or five hours of their shift to become fully involved in any meaningful therapeutic activity, and this in itself limits the effectiveness of the present evening activities provided for patients. The fact that the two-day shifts never overlap has serious disadvantages for continuity of care and the development of ward policies, as well as making it difficult for time to be found for providing any formal teaching for learners and in-service trainees. We understand that the General Nursing Council have in any case recommended, on their visits in 1971 and 1975, that learners should not be required to work the 'long day' shift.

CHAPTER 11

THE MALE BLOCK WARDS

11.1 The physical environment

11.1.1　Patterns of care within a hospital are influenced to some extent by architecture, and Rampton is no exception. The central high security area, with its three-storeyed blocks of wards, now nearly 70 years old, and its long narrow and forbidding connecting corridors, is not dissimilar in style and layout to many older NHS psychiatric hospitals. It reflects the custodial and authoritarian regimes characteristic of most of these hospitals when they were first built. The overall impression is intensified by the heavy internal doors whose constant unlocking and re-locking is a necessary accompaniment of all movement round the hospital. The whole hospital is however in excellent decorative order, and in some areas imaginative re-decoration has gone some way towards lightening the generally rather oppressive atmosphere, although we feel there is scope for further improvements.

11.1.2　Several of the male blocks have recently been redecorated and all are spotlessly clean. They nevertheless present a stark appearance. This is to some extent because of their design; many of the side rooms are narrow and high, giving an unfortunate cell-like impression. But we think much more could be done to improve the physical environment of the wards even given the architectural constraints. There are very few pictures or posters on the walls of common living areas of the wards. Dormitories often have attractive bedspreads and curtains, but no use is made of the pin-boards which are provided for posters, photographs and pictures. Patients are not encouraged to personalise their bed space. What can be done is demonstrated in one particular male block ward (Concord). Pin and thread pictures made by staff and patients, as well as contemporary posters, break up the monotony of the high walls, and there are many potted plants (freely available from the hospital garden) on plant stands around the ward.

11.1.3　One of the criticisms which can be made of the present building layout is that there are insufficient rooms for small group sessions or informal meetings, and the charge nurse's office is often the only place where private interviews can be held. There is an urgent need to improve facilities for private interviews which could probably be met by converting one or more side rooms for the purpose. We understand that a start has already been made on this. The position is even worse on the villas—see paragraph 14.3.2. A reduced patient population should make improvements in this area easier to achieve.

11.1.4　Arguments based on security considerations are frequently used by the staff to justify what we think is an unacceptably low level of physical amenity in the male block wards. There should be a minimum standard which should reflect current perceptions of what is reasonable. No agreed standard exists and current practice sets the threshold at too low a level. We do not think there is justification for the present universal practice in the wards whereby no patients are allowed to have furniture (other than a bed), pictures or personal possessions in their bedrooms. We accept that there may be a

51

minority of disturbed and destructive patients for whom such a rule is necessary, but we think it should be quite exceptional. To give another example, we do not think it right to refuse to allow all male patients on the block wards the use of transistor radios in bed (as at present) just because in the past a patient or patients have tried to strangle themselves with the earpiece cord or have produced sparks from batteries with the object of lighting cigarettes or causing fires.

11.2 Ward regimes

11.2.1 We have already given an account, in the Annex to Part I, of patients' daily routine on the male block wards and the regime to which they are subject. We would like at this stage to draw attention to general features of those regimes where we think changes need to be made.

11.2.2 Firstly, the regime on the wards tends to institutionalise patients and suppress their individuality to an unacceptable degree. We recognise that this is something which is bound to happen to some extent in all 'total institutions', such as boarding schools, long-stay hospitals and prisons. We also recognise that the anti-social and violent tendencies of some Rampton patients on admission may be such that there can be no question at the outset of allowing them much freedom of choice and of self-expression. Nevertheless we think that some nursing practices on the male block wards go too far in the opposite direction. We think that more importance should be attached to patients' having personal possessions more readily accessible to them. For example, although most wards now have larger lockers, on at least two wards patients have to be content with a locker on the ward corridor of less than $3\frac{1}{2}$ cubic feet in volume for all their personal possessions. They are not allowed to keep personal items in their bedrooms or dormitories. Although patients can wear their own clothes, those who have to rely on hospital ones do not have personal issues of shirts or underwear, and may get different ones each week. (We recommend specifically in paragraph 28.6.2 that this practice should be ended.) Razors and razor blades are shared between several patients. On some wards, cleaning the ward is given priority over shaving, so patients do not shave until lunchtime. We were all disturbed by the undignified way in which patients are required to stand together in the corridor whilst changing from day to night clothes and vice versa (although we appreciate that some patients may need close supervision whilst dressing and undressing to ensure that they are not secreting dangerous objects on their persons). Similarly we found the way in which bread and tea are served at meal times objectionable. We think these and similar practices should be re-examined.

11.2.3 Secondly, we draw attention to the almost military insistence on conformity to strict disciplinary rules. We accept that unless there is a proper degree of discipline in an institution like Rampton, internal security is bound to be put at risk. Nevertheless, we question whether it is necessary for example for patients to have to wear ties at all times, to be discouraged from talking at mealtimes or to have to ask permission of a nurse before being allowed to re-enter the dayroom after lighting a cigarette. We think rules of this nature discourage patients from developing self-awareness and self-control and cannot have any usefulness in developing socially acceptable patterns of behaviour. Many of the standards they reflect are in any case not current in the community at large.

11.2.4   We are glad that following staff consultations in September 1980 most of the practices mentioned in the two preceding paragraphs are, we are told, being terminated or reviewed.

11.2.5   Many of the features of the régime on the male block wards on which we have commented are reflections of how the staff on those ward see their role and their attitude towards their patients. We discuss staff attitudes in more detail in Chapter 18.

CHAPTER 12

THE FEMALE BLOCK WARDS

12.1   Female patients constitute about a quarter of the Rampton population. As we pointed out in Chapter 2, they differ significantly from the male
patients in that about 60 per cent are mentally handicapped or severely
handicapped (compared with only about a third of the men), and only 25 per
cent have been admitted following a conviction (compared with 60 per cent of
the males). Our impression is that overall the female population at Rampton
presents even more difficult nursing and general management problems than
the male. Many female patients are very seriously disturbed and violent.
There are frequent attempts, sometimes bizarre, at suicide or self-mutilation,
for example by swallowing such objects as cutlery or attempting self-strangu-
lation using ligatures extracted from sanitary pads. Many patients indulge in
a wide range of other forms of manipulative and attention-seeking behaviour.
The use of tranquillizers and other psychoropic drugs as well as the incidence
of seclusion—see Chapter 13—is substantially higher on the female side of the
hospital than on the male; this is however a commonly observed phenomenon
in psychiatric hospitals generally.

12.2   Apart from the admission ward (see Chapter 9.2) and the high
security special care unit (see paragraph 13.2.5) there are four female block
wards. The architecture and layout described in paragraphs 11.1.1 and 11.1.3
apply equally to the female wards, and the daily routines are in outline similar
to those on the male wards. There are nevertheless very noticeable differences
between the atmosphere and nursing style on the male and female wards.
Overall there is much less regimentation and much more flexibility on the
female side. Observation, though sustained, is much more subtle and generally
the rapport between the staff and patients is much better than on the male
wards. Daily body and bedroom searches are not carried out and searches are
only undertaken if security is threatened because an implement is missing or
if a particular individual is suspect. Differences such as those are symbolically
reflected in the fact that female nurses wear traditional nursing uniform with
a cap and apron, rather than the prison officer style uniform worn by the men.
(We discuss the question of uniform further in Chapter 18.) It is not unusual
to hear patients addressing female ward staff (including some ward sisters) by
Christian or pet names; this would be unthinkable on the male side, even on
a villa. On most female wards staff and patients take great pride in creating a
homely environment. Most wards have been recently redecorated and plants,
floral decorations, posters and ornaments are in evidence everywhere. Day
areas, though often lacking in space, are brightly furnished and carpeted and
patients have more freedom in the use of these areas, including access to the
ward sister's office. Bathrooms and washrooms however are very stark in
appearance and because of size and design afford little privacy for patients.
As on the male side, there are some side rooms where the only furniture is a
bed, but there are other more fully furnished bedrooms and patients are
allowed to have certain possessions in with them, such as handbags, books
and dolls. We noticed other examples of a more flexible approach to routine
characteristic of the female block wards; bedrooms are sometimes opened up

informally after lunch or tea to allow patients who want to lie down on their beds for a few minutes to do so, and patients are not hurried out of the dining-room into the day-room after meals as they tend to be on the male block ward. Female patients do not in general have to do the heavier cleaning jobs on the ward which form part of the daily routine for male block ward patients (although some female wards retain a traditional 'ward worker'). Domestics are employed for most of the heavier work: patient's duties are restricted to tidying their own rooms and making their beds (if fit to do so) and doing small chores like cleaning and laying tables, dusting and plant-watering.

12.3   In general we have no specific criticisms to make of the regime on the female block wards (though the criticisms we make in Chapter 10 of the organisation of the patients' day apply just as much to the female as to the male wards). We have some comments however about the staffing level on one particular ward, Victoria.

12.4   Victoria Ward houses the most severely handicapped female patients; the average occupancy is about 17. They present some peculiarly difficult and intractable nursing problems. The patients are all highly destructive and many have propensities towards self-mutilation. Some will smear their excrement over the floors, walls, and ceilings of the ward; all these surfaces have to be regularly steam-cleaned. Most of the patients cannot be given nightdresses or bedclothes and have to sleep naked under strong untearable rugs on mattresses on the floor.

12.5   The ward has recently been redecorated and the furniture in the day-room has been upholstered in specially strong material. The day areas in general are of necessity sparsely furnished and the few pictures and decorations hang well above eye level out of harm's way.

12.6   We were greatly impressed by the kindness and dedication of the nursing staff on Victoria, doing a job which few people would find it easy to undertake. In our view however the day time nursing complement of seven is far too low for this type of unit. The staff are stretched to the limit in coping with the difficult behavioural problems of their patients and this leaves no time for them to teach or train their patients to any significant degree. We were particularly concerned about the situation first thing in the morning, when the inadequate number of nurses have to share with their patients in all the indignities of cleaning side rooms, emptying chamber pots, disposing of soiled linen and herding patients to the toilet areas to be washed and dressed. In the evening patients have at times to be locked in their rooms as early as 6.00 pm, which means that they are effectively cut off from any form of social or therapeutic activity for 14 hours at a stretch. Inadequate staff ratios mean that it is difficult to create a therapeutic atmosphere on the ward and that patients therefore tend to respond to the disturbed behaviour of their fellow patients, thus perpetuating their behavioural problems.

12.7   We are seriously concerned about the situation on this ward, and we think that urgent action should be taken to remedy it. We think that the aim should be to separate the patients into family size groups with a true staff ratio of at least 1:1 throughout the working day. Nursing staff changes should be kept to a minimum and all the regular ward staff should be given the opportunity to attend courses and seminars on behaviour modification techniques. At the earliest opportunity an individual re-assessment of each patient should be made in consultation with a clinical psychologist, and an individual programme agreed, with each patient's progress being carefully and regularly monitored. These recommendations could equally well apply to most wards of the hospital but we consider that the situation in Victoria Ward commands the highest priority.

CHAPTER 13

HANDLING DISTURBED AND VIOLENT BEHAVIOUR

13.1   As one would expect, disturbed and violent patient behaviour is common at Rampton. Isolated and trivial incidents of bad behaviour or rule-breaking (many of which would hardly count as violent or disturbed behaviour) are dealt with informally by nursing staff, whether by admonition, temporary withdrawal of privileges (such as attendance at social functions), extra domestic work or 'fining' through the points system (see paragraph 23.1.4). In more serious cases, where the patient's behaviour constitutes a continuing threat to the safety of himself, other patients or staff, the patient may have to be 'secluded', ie temporarily confined to a side room. When there is continuing disturbed or violent behaviour, the patient may need transfer to a high security 'special care' unit—what used to be called a 'refractory ward'—Drake Ward for men, Alexandra Ward for women.

13.2   Seclusion

13.2.1   Seclusion means locking a patient in a side room (usually one specially designated for the purpose) during the daytime. The rules currently in force at Rampton provide that the side room doors should be opened for 'feeding, exercise, and medication' for three half-hour periods in the course of the day.

13.2.2   Seclusion is authorised by the nurse in charge of the ward, who has to record the reason for the action in the ward report and in the patient's clinical file. The duty doctor (and the patient's consultant, if he is on duty) and the nursing officer in charge of the unit have to be informed immediately, but there is no requirement that they should visit the patient straightaway. They are however required to visit the patient daily. The patient must be visited at least once every 15 minutes by the ward staff.

13.2.3   When a patient is secluded, it is a common practice to give an intra-muscular injection of a phenothiazine drug (a major tranquilizer). If the phenothiazine has already been prescribed p.r.n. (*'pro re nata'*—'as and when required'), this injection can be given without reference to a doctor.

13.2.4   Some patients are on 'voluntary' seclusion, that is, they ask to be secluded because, for example, they feel unable to control their own aggression. Although statistics are not readily available, our impression is that on the male side of the hospital voluntary seclusion may represent as much as a third of all incidents. The procedures used (often including a phenothiazine injection) are the same as for the compulsory seclusion.

13.2.5   Seclusion is recorded far more frequently for female patients than for male. We looked at the figures for three separate months in 1979, and found that on any one day between seven per cent and nine per cent of the female population were likely to be secluded, compared with under one per cent of the men.

57

13.2.6   The Rampton rules on seclusion to which we have referred say that 'the period of seclusion must be kept to the minimum commensurate with safety'. Seclusion however not infrequently lasts for quite extended periods, and indeed a small number of patients of necessity are in more or less permanent seclusion, for example, some severely mentally handicapped female patients.

13.2.7   We accept that seclusion will at times be necessary to cope with the behaviour of the more seriously disturbed patients at Rampton. We think the formal rules for controlling and monitoring its use are by and large satisfactory and we have no reason to believe that they are not fully complied with by the staff. Nor have we any evidence which suggests that seclusion is over-used or used in cases where it is clearly inappropriate. A slightly revised and expanded version of the formal rules is at present under discussion within the hospital. We note with approval that the draft revised procedure makes it clear that the primary (we would prefer to say the only) function of seclusion is the removal of the severely disturbed patient from potential danger to himself ot others, that it is to be clearly distinguished from 'time out from positive reinforcement' under a planned behaviour modification programme, and that it is not to be used as a punitive measure.

13.2.8   We think nevertheless that there are various questions about the use of seclusion which Rampton staff ought to consider. When a patient becomes violent or disturbed, seclusion is an obvious and effective short-term measure. But it may do little if anything to deal with the underlying cause of the patient's violent behaviour or help his progress in the longer term. Physical restraint, of which seclusion is one form, can never be more than a short-term palliative for disturbed behaviour by someone who is mentally disturbed, and we think it is important that staff should always bear in mind that in the longer term there may be alternative ways of controlling or preventing violence. In our view after every incident of seclusion the medical and nursing staff concerned should discuss the events to try and ascertain why the patient became violent and whether those factors which trigger off violence can be reduced and ways found of helping to control aggressive behaviour in future. The widely different usage rate of seclusion on the male and female sides of the hospital might bear some investigation in this context; it seems to us possible that seclusion, together with the staff attention and extra medication associated with it, may be positively sought by disturbed female patients as a way of acquiring status amongst their peers.

13.2.9   We have three other specific recommendations on seclusion. First, there should in our view rarely be any need for an injection when a patient is secluded voluntarily; oral medication should generally be sufficient in such cases. Secondly, the rules should provide for early visits by doctors to secluded patients and not just, as at present, for them to be informed and for a visit to be made within 24 hours. Thirdly, we think it is important that senior nurse management should always have a complete and up-to-date picture of the extent to which seclusion is being used (including the length of time any particular patient has been secluded), and that the system of recording seclusion should be reviewed to achieve this aim.

13.3 Special care units

13.3.1   If a patient shows continuing disturbed or violent behaviour he may be transferred to one of the high security special care units—Drake Ward for men, Alexandra Ward for women. The period individual patients spend on these wards can vary between a few days to, exceptionally, in the case of the most disturbed patients, months or even years. We are told that most new female admissions have a spell on Alexandra; like seclusion (see 13.2.8 above), it may be something of a 'status symbol'.

13.3.2   Both special care units have a higher staff/patient ratio than that of the other block wards. The standard of physical security is also exceptionally high.

13.3.3   The principal differences between the routine on Drake Ward and that in the other male block wards are directly related to the increased need to observe all patients constantly to prevent aggression or self-injury. On waking, all patients are closely examined; the bedclothes are also searched even more carefully than on other block wards and the blankets and bed linen are folded into a pack. Patients do not handle razors and shaving is performed by the nursing staff. Cleaning occupies the whole morning period and is performed to a standard usually seen only in operating theatres. Walls as well as floors are washed and the day-room is polished with old-fashioned bumpers. Corridor and bedroom floors receive most attention and patients clean them daily on their hands and knees. Patients do not attend the occupations department or other hospital activities but provided their physical and mental condition permits they are kept active within the ward or its adjacent airing court. There is ward occupational therapy during the afternoons, consisting of simple contract work performed without tools. A spell on the airing court and TV viewing are the main social diversions; a bonus at the weekend is the opportunity to watch hospital football.

13.3.4   There are significant differences, between the regime on Drake Ward and that on Alexandra Ward, the equivalent female ward. On Alexandra there is far more interaction between patients and staff. Whilst domestic tasks are allocated to all, much more emphasis is placed on light occupational and recreational therapy organised by the ward nurses. As an incentive to good behaviour patients are permitted to attend social functions for block ward patients. All these examples reflect the general difference in nursing style between the male and female sides of the hospital which we discussed in the previous chapter.

13.3.5   Work is well advanced on constructing a new special treatment unit for 20 acutely disturbed female patients. This involves the radical reconstruction of one of the other female block wards (Catherine). It is hoped that this unit can be brought into commission early next year. It will accommodate the patients at present on Alexandra Ward and it is hoped that it may also be able to take a small number af disturbed severely mentally handicapped patients from Victoria Ward (see paragraphs 12.4–7 above).

13.3.6   If the changes we advocate for the block wards can be applied to the special care units we see no need to make specific recommendations for those units. There may be need to modify the changes in the light of the special circumstances of those units, but we think it important that the standard of amenity on them and the degree of flexibility in treatment programmes for individual patients should be as high as possible consistent with the safety of patients and staff.

CHAPTER 14

THE VILLAS

14.1   Patients usually spend two or three years on the block wards. When they are judged ready to move out into the villas, their pattern of life undergoes a significant change.

14.2   Most of the 19 villa wards were built in the 1930s as detached two storey units situated at varying distances from each other in well-kept gardens. All the villas are within the outer security area, except the two male pre-discharge villas, Moss Rose and Sweet Briar, which are outside the main fence altogether but have their own fences enclosing the villa ward gardens. Five villas are specialised units dealing with elderly patients and the more severely mentally handicapped male and female patients. The ten non-specialist male villas fall into three categories, preliminary, preparatory and pre-discharge, and patients progressing through the 'system' (see paragraph 7.1.2 will normally spend some time in a villa of each type. There are only two non-specialist female villas of which Poplars is preparatory and Linden is pre-discharge.

14.3   The preliminary, preparatory and pre-discharge villas

14.3.1   Villa patients sleep in single rooms and dormitories as in the block wards and are locked into their rooms at night. As they move towards the pre-discharge stage however, they appear to have more access to their rooms during the evening and are able to keep more personal possessions there. Male patients are for the first time able to personalise their rooms with pictures and posters. Lavatories and showers are usually left open all day, so patients have unrestricted access to them. There are usually two day-rooms, one with TV, the other with stereo, table tennis, darts and patients' lockers. Many of these rooms, particularly in the pre-discharge villas, are attractively decorated and furnished. Patients play a more active part in serving food than on the block wards, and the catering arrangements are much less formal.

14.3.2.   The shortage of private interview rooms which we noted on the block wards (paragraph 11.1.3) is even more marked on the villas. We hope ways can be found of remedying this.

14.3.3   Villa patients have more social privileges than block ward patients. There are social evenings arranged specifically for them, and much more opportunities to take part in organised games and various inter-villa competitions. There are also annual outings to the seaside and to Clumber Park, a local beauty spot. As discharge gets nearer supervised employment outside the hospital perimeter increases, and there are shopping trips to local towns once a month. Progress through the villas is reflected in less formal dress for male patients; hairstyles also become more individual and beards may be grown.

14.3.4   The style of nursing in the villas, at any rate on the male side, is markedly different in many ways from that in the block wards. Social distance between staff and patients is less apparent, and patients are more often addressed by their Christian names. Although the staff/patient ratio is only just over half that in the block wards, nurses seem to be able to find much more time for a game of darts or table tennis, and patients appear to feel more free to approach staff both in or out of the ward office. Morale and general atmosphere in many villas is clearly very good.

14.3.5   There are some excellent multi-disciplinary and other programmes available to patients in the villas. For example, we were impressed by programmes provided by Team 1 on Oaks Ward (preparatory) where there are social advisory groups, self-catering courses, and a doctor-led patient discussion group. On the female side there are similar social advisory groups; we also liked the self-contained flatlet on Linden Ward, where two patients at a time can learn to look after and budget for themselves in quite realistic circumstances (except that they are not allowed to handle cash—see paragraph 15.4). We would like to see a similar facility provided if posible on the two male predischarge villas, Moss Rose and Sweet Briar.

14.4   Villas for the elderly

Juniper (male) and Larch (female) house long-term elderly patients, many of whom have known no other home. (Larch also takes physically ill female villa patients.) Although lacking the freedon and outings that a comparable group of NHS elderly mentally infirm patients would enjoy, in other respects their quality of life is not dissimilar.

14.5   The specialist mental handicap villas

14.5.1   Rowans, Hollies and Maples are the three specialist mental handicap villas. Rowans takes the low dependency male patients. The quality of care afforded is impressive, and the environment good; there is a variety of occupational and diversional therapy, and all 'activity group' opportunities (see Chapter 21) are used to the full.

14.5.2   Hollies and Maples Wards take the more highly dependent male and female patients respectively. Hollies accommodates 30 male patients and Maples 24 female patients. These patients require a higher rate of staff to provide the basic care to meet personal needs and to cope with the severe behaviour problems. In both villas, episodes of violence towards other patients and staff, destruction of clothing and property, and self-injury or self-mutilation are common. The care and training programmes for the patients are of a high standard, and there are satisfactory levels of dedicated and experienced staff. They face however some special problems in tackling their already difficult task. The design of the wards is unsuitable for this kind of patient; the creation of a home-like environment in a large two-storey building is very difficult. In the case of Hollies, a reduction in patient numbers to 20–25 would help to allow more individual care and attention. The scarcity of clinical psychologists, to which we have alluded in several other parts of our report, has inhibited the development of the more sophisticated forms of treatment such as individual behaviour modification programmes. Moreover, the development of self-help skills is hampered by the rigidity of the day-to-day routine of the institution. Staff have insufficient time, particularly in the morning, for helping patients to do things for themselves rather than doing things for them.

Similar problems arise on the specialist mentally handicapped block wards. An earlier start to the day seems the most obvious answer, but this would seem to depend on changes in the nurses' shift system (see Chapter 10).

14.5.3   Many patients in the wards described in this section have been pronounced suitable for transfer to a NHS hospital. We discuss the problem of transfer in the next chapter.

14.6   Conclusions

Overall and subject to the points made above we were impressed with the villa wards and the work being done in them. The lay-out of the buildings is however clearly now in many ways out-dated in the light of modern nursing ideas, and we hope that at least one more modern unit can be provided as soon as possible.

CHAPTER 15

DISCHARGE AND TRANSFER

15.1 By statute special hospitals are provided for persons who 'in [the Secretary of State's] opinion require treatment under conditions of special security'. When a patient's condition has improved to the extent that he no longer requires treatment in Rampton, it is in everyone's interest that he should leave as soon as possible and, if he still requires treatment, receive it elsewhere. Detention in a special hospital will always represent a grave restriction on a patient's individual freedom, and it is quite wrong that anyone should be subject to it longer than necessary.

15.2 Rampton's 1972 hospital policy document (see Appendix D) is based on the assumption that most Rampton patients can respond to treatment and rehabilitation to such an extent that they can eventually, after a greater or lesser period of time, be made fit for life outside Rampton, preferably in the community but alternatively in some other sort of institution. We entirely endorse this assumption, and what happens in practice shows that it is not an unrealistic one. It appears that most patients do in fact eventually leave Rampton. We agree with the 1972 document that the main aim of Rampton's therapeutic and rehabilitation policies should be to prepare patients for discharge or transfer (henceforth in this chapter, for the sake of brevity, 'departure') as soon as possible.

15.3 We have found it convenient to consider departure under three separate aspects: how patients are prepared for departure, how they are selected for departure and how decisions that a patient should depart are put into effect.

15.4 Preparation for departure

Despite much good work, notably in the occupations and education departments, we do not think that the avowed aim of Rampton's rehabilitation policy, to prepare patients for eventual departure, is adequately reflected in many of the actual practices at Rampton. As we have indicated, we think that many features of the nursing regime, particularly on the male block wards, give patients little opportunity to develop the self-reliance, the sound skills and the self-awareness and self-control which they will need to be able to cope with life outside a highly structured institutional framework. The position is clearly a lot better on the villas, but here too there is room for improvement. We think that more thought should be given to programmes designed to give realistic practice in dealing with situations likely to arise in the outside world. We commend the development of a more flexible and less uniform security regime, as suggested in Chapter 8.6. We think that the experimental pre-discharge group home training unit temporarily housed in the old Moss Rose school should be extended and continued; we accept that this will involve a different venue because of the decision which has already been taken by the Rampton Policy Committee to set up a patients' workshop on that site. This latter decision should be implemented forthwith (see paragraph 23.4.2). The rehabilitative function of the patients' shop needs urgent review (see paragraph

28.8.3); in particular we think ways should be found of allowing at least pre-departure patients to use cash in the shop. Outside shopping trips for pre-discharge patients should be encouraged and extended.

15.5 Selection for departure

15.5.1 The procedure for deciding when a patient is fit for departure can vary considerably from case to case depending largely on the patient's legal status. 'Unrestricted' patients can be discharged at any time, by the RMO, (the patient's 'responsible medical officer' under the Mental Health Act, ie the consultant in charge of his case) a MHRT, or (in certain very rare circumstances) by the patient's nearest relative. DHSS have to approve proposals by a RMO for transfer of an unrestricted patient to a NHS hospital. Discharges or transfer of restricted patients have to be approved by the Home Secretary, who in appropriate cases consults his Advisory Board on Restricted Patients (the 'Aarvold Board'). We refer in paragraph 5.13.2 to the delays which sometimes arise at this stage and think that urgent steps should be taken to remedy them. Otherwise we think the procedures on the whole work reasonably well, given the structure of the Mental Health Act (which is at present under review by the Government).

15.5.2 We are, of course, aware that there have been cases where subsequent tragic events have shown that the decision to discharge or transfer a particular patient was, in the light of hindsight, a wrong one. Such instances are rare and we believe inevitable simply because it is impossible to make correct predictions about future behaviour in every case, however careful the system. It is better to accept this inevitability than to condemn all patients to permanent custody within special hospitals. At the hospital level we think the best safeguard against wrong decisions is for RMOs regularly to seek the professional advice of colleagues in other disciplines before deciding whether or not to recommend that a patient should depart, and this is usually what happens at Rampton. Indeed we would go further, and refrain from criticizing (as some who have given us their view have invited us to do) those RMOs who advise their patients to apply to MHRTs for a decision to discharge, rather than taking the decision themselves; other things being equal, it is probably always better to share responsibility for a decision in this sort of case.

15.5.3 Under the provisions of the Mental Health Act, (or, in the case of 'restricted' patients, as a matter of administrative practice) a detained patient's case must be reviewed after the first year of detention and then every two years. This should ensure that those suitable for discharge or transfer are not overlooked. We are satisfied that this review is properly carried out at Rampton under the control of the medical records department.

15.5.4 We should mention at this stage that as part of our review we arranged for all the mentally handicapped patients at Rampton to be assessed in December 1979 using the Wessex mental handicap register form. This survey produced data on each patient's basic level of self-care, mobility, communication and literacy skills and also on the frequency and severity of problem behaviours. The data suggests at first sight that there may be more mentally handicapped patients suitable for discharge or transfer from Rampton than appear on the official waiting list. However this can only be a tentative view without a detailed case-by-case clinical review of each of the patients concerned by staff at the hospital. We have accordingly arranged for all the data from our survey to be sent to Rampton for further action on these lines.

15.6   Putting decisions to discharge or transfer into effect

15.6.1   Once a decision has been taken that a patient is ready to depart, it does not unfortunately follow that this will happen within a reasonable period. It may prove difficult to find anywhere suitable for him to go to. It became clear to us at an early stage of our work that this aspect of departure presented peculiarly intractable problems.

15.6.2   In recent years, of the annual departures from Rampton (119 in 1979), just over a third have been discharges, principally by decision of the Mental Health Review Tribunal. The majority of departures have been transfers to NHS hospitals. Expressed as a proportion of the total hospital population, Rampton's annual departure rate has risen from 13 per cent in 1970 to 15 per cent in 1979, although these figures do not tell the whole story (see paragraph 15.6.4 below).

15.6.3   We look first at transfers. Of those a substantial proportion have been to the Eastdale Unit at Balderton Hospital, near Newark. This Unit was opened in 1974, specifically for male ex-special hospital (particularly Rampton) patients. At present it takes up to 12 patients at a time, for a maximum of six months. The aim is that patients accepted for Eastdale should at the end of that period be ready for discharge direct into the community. Eastdale does not take severely mentally handicapped patients. Eastdale's contribution to the improvement in the annual departure rate has been a substantial one. We understand that the future of the Unit is at present under review. We firmly recommend that it should be retained and that provision be made for it to take more patients from Rampton (as we understand may be possible if more staff can be provided). We also think that the possibility of providing a similar unit for female patients should be explored.

15.6.4   But the crucial problem at Rampton (which the improvement in the overall annual departure rate conceals) is finding a place for these patients who no longer need to be kept in a special hospital but who are not fit for discharge and whom Eastdale, for one reason or another (eg because they are severely mentally handicapped or need long-term hospital care) cannot take. On 1 July 1980 there were 122 patients at Rampton on the 'waiting-list' for transfer (including transfer to Eastdale). Of these 92 (75 per cent) had been on the list for over six months, and 51 (42 per cent) for over two years. Of those waiting over six months, 57 (62 per cent) were classified as subnormal or severely subnormal; of those waiting over two years, 41 (71 per cent) were so classified. The most intractable waiting-list problem at Rampton is finding places for patients who need transferring to NHS mental handicap hospitals.

15.6.5   It is possible that the projected regional secure units (RSUs) will, when they are operational, help alleviate the problem, by providing accommodation for some patients transferred from special hospitals for whom suitable 'medium secure' accommodation would not otherwise be available. Much will depend on the clinical policies adopted by individual units, but it seems at this stage doubtful whether they will have very much to offer to severely mentally handicapped patients or those requiring treatment in secure conditions for a long period of time. In any case, it is clearly going to be several years before a significant number of RSU places are available, and we do not think any reliance should be placed on them as a possible partial solution for Rampton's problem in the short or indeed the medium-term.

15.6.6   The DHSS have themselves recognised the problem for some time, and, before we were set up, had commissioned a research project on the problems of transferring patients from special hospitals generally to NHS hospitals. This research was undertaken by Mrs Susanne Dell, whose report has now been published*. As we do, she indentifies the difficulty of finding places in mental handicap hospitals as the dominant feature of the whole transfer problem. She describes the two ways in which NHS places are sought for special hospital patients: the 'formal' method whereby DHSS, as managers of the hospital, are asked to find a place and to approach the Regional Health Authority responsible for the patient's home area; and the 'informal' method whereby a special hospital consultant approaches a medical colleague in a particular hospital. She finds that the 'informal method' has proved significantly more effective in placing mentally handicapped patients than the 'formal method', particularly if the 'receiving' consultant can be persuaded to visit the patient at the special hospital. She describes how lack of room is the most common reason given by mental handicap hospitals for not taking ex-special hospital patients, and suggests that the transfer problems of mentally handicapped special hospital patients are largely a reflection of inadequate services currently available for the mentally handicapped generally. She suggests that special hospitals should make more use of the 'informal method' and should consider whether conditional discharge, to a hostel or into the community, could be an acceptable alternative for some patients on the waiting-list for transfer.

15.6.7   We commend these proposals as far as they lie within our terms of reference, but we note that Rampton's waiting-list for transfer could be reduced by a third if the backlog of mentally handicapped patients who have been on it for more than two years were cleared. We think this particular group of patients should receive special priority, and that a joint effort should be made urgently by Rampton and the NHS, with the help of DHSS, to find places for them. We would expect the medical staff at Rampton to take the lead on this, and suggest it should be high on the new Medical Director's list of priorities (see paragraph 16.7.6 below).

15.6.8   We have two other suggestions which we think may help the transfer problem. First, we think that the more Rampton consultants are involved in the procedure for admitting patients particularly those admitted from NHS hospitals—see paragraph 9.1.4—the more links they will form with NHS hospitals and the easier they will find it to get patients transferred. Secondly,

*Special Hospitals Research Report No 16. The Transfer of Special Hospital Patients to National Health Service hospitals, by Susanne Dell. DHSS 1980.

67

and more generally, we think that Rampton has a poor image in the NHS. The Yorkshire TV programme and other unfavourable publicity has given NHS staff an excuse to be unwilling to receive ex-Rampton patients. If in the light of our recommendations elsewhere in this report, Rampton can become a better place it will get a better reputation and this will make it easier to get its ex-patients accepted.

15.7 So far as discharge is concerned, the main difficulty is the (understandable) unwillingness of some local authorities social services departments to give financial priority to and so make available scarce and expensive hostel places for ex-Rampton patients, particularly those who may not have lived in their area for many years. One possible solution to this problem would be for Rampton itself to set up hostels for its ex-patients. Whilst we would not wish positively to discourage efforts in this direction, we suspect that any proposal for a hostel which was labelled as being exclusively or mainly for ex-Rampton patients would meet with such resistance from the local community that the scheme would have great difficulty in getting off the ground. In our view a more promising way forward would be for DHSS to extend the present arrangements whereby it can make extra-statutory payments to maintain for six months a limited number of ex-special hospital patients in local authority hostels. These arrangements might be extended to hostels run by voluntary organisations.

CHAPTER 16

THE MEDICAL STAFF

16.1   At the time of writing the full-time medical staff in post at Rampton comprises eight consultants and five medical assistants. An additional consultant post has been authorised but no appointment has yet been made. There is a part-time consultant psychotherapist and nine clinical assistant (general practitioner) sessions are provided each week.

16.2   The Consultants

16.2.1   The consultants bear full clinical responsibility for patients under their care and each consultant is designated as a responsible medical officer (RMO) under the provisions of the Mental Health Act 1959.

16.2.2   Recruitment of consultants at Rampton has never been easy and there are almost always vacancies to be filled and a considerable turnover of locum appointments. There are a number of reasons for this. The nature of the work does not appeal to many; the constraints imposed upon the consultants' powers to admit or discharge (see paragraphs 9.1.1 and 15.5.1) may appear irksome to some, and the lack of out-patient work or community and domiciliary involvement makes posts less attractive than in the NHS mental health service. The long-term nature of much of the clinical work, the frustrations of the all-pervading security dimension, and the onerous responsibility of decision-taking in regard to an individual patient where an error of judgement might have disastrous consequences, all combine to make the position of the special hospital consultant a singularly "special" one. There are also financial disadvantages because of the lack of opportunities for private work and domiciliary visits which are available to other consultants in psychiatry. Added to these difficulties is Rampton's geographical remoteness and professional isolation both of which increase its unattractiveness to doctors.

16.2.3   We think that a shortage of suitable applicants for consultant posts has undoubtedly led in the past to some appointments being made on the grounds of expediency rather than suitability but efforts have been made in recent years to raise the threshold of qualifications, training and experience. Candidates for appointment have for some time been formally interviewed by a committee which includes an assessor nominated by the Royal College of Psychiatrists. All but one of the consultants now in post hold post-graduate specialist qualifications in psychiatry and have had experience in psychiatric hospitals or the prison medical service. The remaining consultant has worked as a locum at Rampton for the past six years and has had considerable psychiatric experience, although he has no formal post-graduate qualification.

16.2.4   We think it is essential that Rampton should be able to attract and retain medical staff of a high calibre. If medical staff who are able and willing to provide leadership and guidance in matters of treatment and care are to be encouraged to work at Rampton, despite the unattractive features of the work which we have mentioned, some positive incentives must be provided. The hospital should be able to offer better clinical facilities, particularly in the field of clinical psychology (see Chapter 25), in order to improve the range of available care and to encourage the development of special interests and research. Financial recognition is also important. Medical staff in the special hospitals recently began receiving the lead payment that has for some time been enjoyed by other categories of staff over their counterparts elsewhere in the NHS (see paragraph 2.6.3). We think it reasonable that in addition an appropriate fee should be negotiated for RMOs' reports to, and appearances before, MHRTs. This work already takes up a high proportion of their time. It will increase even further if there is a shortening of the statutory review periods for patients compulsorily detained under the Mental Health Act, as advocated in current proposals.

16.2.5 We think it is important to take steps to lessen the professional isolation of doctors at Rampton. The movement of consultants between the special hospitals should be encouraged, with appropriate upset and removal expenses being paid. All other possibilities for broadening experience and training should be thoroughly explored: these might include the greater use of proleptic appointments (that is, appointments coming into effect some time after they are actually made, to enable the person appointed to get experience elsewhere first), encouragement to take sabbaticals and study leave with pay and expenses, both at home and abroad, and perhaps, as the HAS suggested in 1971, joint appointments with other NHS hospitals and academic centres.

16.2.6 The consultants at Rampton are each responsible for the care of some 100 patients. The number of consultant posts has gradually risen over the past decade, reflecting an increase in the level of clinical activity at the hospital. It has been put to us that the number of consultant posts should be increased still further because the staff/patient ratio is still low compared with other special hospitals. In view of the likely difficulties, at any rate in the short term, of attracting sufficient suitable candidates we do not think this is a realistic option at the present time. We think the aim should be instead to reduce the overall patient population, which would have the effect of reducing consultants' work load, as well as being desirable on other grounds (see paragraph 5.11). Recruitment of more clinical psychologists (see paragraph 16.2.4 above) could also provide some relief for consultants.

16.2.7 We think it should be borne in mind when consultants are being appointed at Rampton that the medical work in the hospital is by no means exclusively appropriate for specialists in forensic psychiatry. General psychiatrists and specialists in mental handicap also have an important contribution to make. We believe that suitable candidates might be forthcoming in larger numbers if there was this recognition of the broader base of work at Rampton.

16.2.8 We refer elsewhere to the lack of leadership displayed by consultants at Rampton. To a large extent this seems to have arisen from the narrow view of their responsibilities taken by many of those appointed in the past. They saw themselves as having no more than an individual responsibility for the particular patients for whom they were the RMO, an individual responsibility to be jealously guarded against any suggestion that the problems of their patients could usefully be discussed with persons of other disciplines or indeed with other consultants. They rejected any suggestion that the doctors individually or corporately had a role to play in the way the hospital was run or the philosophies of treatment which should be adopted. If Rampton is to make the progress we hope to see, this sort of attitude can have no place in the future.

16.3 Medical assistants

16.3.1 Medical assistants constitute a sub-consultant grade which is being phased out in other parts of the NHS. New appointments to the grade can in general only be made on a personal basis: last year, however, Rampton got special permission from the DHSS Central Manpower Committee to advertise two additional posts in this grade, and these have now been filled, bringing the total number of medical assistants up to five. An application has recently gone to the DHSS for permission to advertise a sixth post.

16.3.2 Medical assistants have been retained at Rampton because of the difficulty of providing appropriate posts for the usual junior training grades (see section 16.6 below) and the consequent need for alternative ways of providing consultants with medical support. They are nominally attached to a consultant's clinical team, but in practice appear to have a large measure of autonomy in their activities and seem to perform many of their duties by 'gentlemen's agreements' amongst themselves. On the male wards of the hospital, they attend to the day-to-day physical care and well-being of the patients; on the female wards, the patients' physical health is looked after by general practitioners from a local practice working sessions as clinical assistants. On both male and female wards, medical assistants become involved to a substantial extent in the treatment of patients' mental as well as physical conditions. They provide an on-call emergency rota for the hospital as a whole, and see patients' relatives, often at weekends.

16.3.3 We feel that there is clearly a need for further discussion towards rationalisation of the role and functions of the medical assistants, with closer involvement with clinical teams wherever possible.

16.4 Psychotherapy

A consultant psychotherapist visits Rampton one day a week from Leicester and sees some individual patients. In addition, two of the consultants have embarked upon a part-time psychotherapy training course at Sheffield University. We think an increased psychotherapy contribution would be a valuable extra treatment resource and could also be helpful in discussion and training groups for nurses and other staff.

16.5 GP clinical assistant sessions

The nine clinical assistant sessions are provided from a local general practice—five of the sessions represent an 'on-call' commitment. As explained above, they cover the physical health of the female patients at the hospital. This appears to work satisfactorily and has the advantage of bringing further contact with the world outside.

16.6 Medical training

16.6.1   In the recent past there have been two medical training posts at the hospital, one for a senior registrar and one optional rotational post for a registrar. The senior registrar post has only had one incumbent (in 1977/78) and remains vacant as it has not been approved fro training by the Joint Committee on Higher Psychiatric Training (JCHPT) who inspected the hospital in December 1978. There are no prospects at present of the post being re-established full-time; we think, however, that it might well form part of a senior registrar training post based elsewhere in the Trent region and that there should be further discussions between the hospital, local universities and the JCHPT to see how this could be achieved.

16.6.2.   The registrar post has been filled for short periods, but has not been recognised for training by the Royal College of Psychiatrists since July 1979. Detailed recommendations were made at that time with a view to eventual re-approval as part of a rotational scheme, but we are doubtful whether a registrar post would be appropriate at present.

16.7   The organisation of medical work at Rampton

16.7.1   Rampton had a Medical Superintendent until 1974. He had management responsibilities for the hospital as a whole (see paragraph 29.2.2). He also had considerable control over the work of the other consultants in the hospital; they were not allowed, for example, to move a patient from a block ward to a villa, or on to an outside working party, without his consent. He had the right to read and comment upon any official reports they made. The other consultants became increasingly unwilling to work to this pattern and insisted upon unfettered individual clinical responsibility for patients under their care.

16.7.2   The Elliott Report in 1973 (see paragraph 3.4 and Appendix F) was critical of the then Medical Superintendent (as well as of the Principal Nursing Officer and the Chief Occupations Officer), and it was decided by DHSS that the post should be abolished. In January 1974, a part-time Medical Director was appointed for a period of two years. He was a consultant based in a mental handicap hospital some 20 miles away, and had no specific clinical responsibilities at Rampton. His function, DHSS have told us, was 'to act in a general administrative capacity and to encourage senior hospital staff of all disciplines to work together and to solve their own problems'. There was a Medical Advisory Committee which included all the Rampton medical staff; its Chairman, a Rampton consultant, represented the Rampton doctors on the Hospital Executive Team, whose Chairman was the Medical Director. A number of highly desirable changes in the organisation of medical work occurred during this time, such as the establishment of consultant clinical teams and case-conferences. The management arrangements as such, however, came under criticism (see paragraph 29.2.4), and the post of Medical Director was allowed to lapse in 1976.

16.7.3   The present management arrangements, described in detail in Chapter 29.2, came into effect soon afterwards. All consultants (and the Chairman of the Medical Advisory Committee, if not a consultant) were to be members of the Hospital Policy Committee, and the Chairman of the Medical

Advisory Committee was also a member of the three-man Hospital Executive Committee.

16.7.4 The subsequent history of the Medical Advisory Committee is an unhappy one, and with the benefit of hindsight it is clear that it was an unwise decision to set up a structure of medical management which provided no proper co-ordinating mechanism and did nothing to encourage the emergence of a leader amongst the medical staff. Continuing clashes of views, philosophies and personalities, sometimes centering around rivalry between the consultants and the medical assistants, led to much discord and bitterness with the result that there were frequent changes of Chairman, no consistent medical participation in management, and an almost total lack of medical leadership. By the early part of 1979 the system of medical representation had broken down altogether with the resignation of the then Chairman and the Vice-Chairman and for a period of over six months there was no medical member on the Hospital Executive Committee. The failure of the medical staff to reach consensus, provide coherent clinical policies, or to contribute effectively to the daily administration of the hospital has resulted in a shift of much of the responsibility for the general running of the hospital to the senior nursing staff.

16.7.5 Since our arrival on the scene in the late autumn of 1979 a Consultants' Committee, with two representatives of the medical assistants, has been established, a chairman elected and a credible medical presence re-established on the Hospital Executive. During the preceding unhappy era however much harm was done to the professional standing and credibility of the medical staff as a group, although it is fair to say that to some extent the medical staff were themselves the victims of the ill-designed system of medical management within which they had to work.

16.7.6 Over the past decade several styles of medical management organisation have been tried and all have proved unsatisfactory for different reasons. At present, following the formation of a Consultants' Advisory Committee with limited medical assistant representation, it has proved possible to elect a Chairman to serve on the Executive. However, the present arrangement cannot be regarded as more than a welcome but temporary development because the present incumbent is near to retirement. We think it vital to provide Rampton with continuing medical leadership and medical participation in management on a more effective basis, and it is our view that this can best be achieved by the establishment of the post of Medical Director. This post would differ in several important respects from the former Medical Director's post which existed between 1974–1976. We think it is essential that the Medical Director should be full-time and that he should have clinical responsibilities as a consultant at Rampton, though these would need to be restricted in size to allow him to devote the majority of his time to his wider commitments. We consider that he should be responsible for devising a system for the allocation of clinical work amongst the medical staff in consultation with his medical colleagues. Although in general consultants would have full clinical autonomy over patients in their care, because of the security dimension at Rampton the Medical Director should be given the right to comment on

73

any report by a consultant recommending discharge, transfer or the granting of leave of absence of any patient.

16.7.7   In addition to his specifically medical duties, we would hope and expect that the Medical Director would provide the overall co-ordination and leadership which Rampton as a whole so much needs. We discuss this further in paragraph 29.4.2.

16.7.8   It will be clear that a doctor of exceptional calibre will be required to fill such a challenging and exacting post, and we think it is essential that the remuneration offered should be such as to attract suitable candidates.

16.7.9   Under our proposals the Chairman of the Medical Advisory Committee would not be concerned with the day-to-day management of the hospital as a whole and the need for a separate Consultants Advisory Committee with only restricted representation of medical assistants would largely disappear. A full Medical Advisory Committee, comprising all hospital medical staff, should be reconstituted and should elect its own Chairman.

CHAPTER 17

OTHER MEDICAL, CLINICAL AND DIAGNOSTIC SERVICES

17.1 Miscellaneous Medical Services

17.1.1   The facilities for physical examination and treatment of patients at Rampton are generally satisfactory. General medical and surgical services appear to function adequately, with access to medical and orthopaedic out-patient clinics at Retford and other services at Worksop Hospital. A full range of pathology and other investigative services is also available at Worksop Hospital. A consultant anaesthetist visits Rampton when ECT is carried out. An ophthalmologist visits regularly. A radiographer pays weekly visits and has the use of a small X-ray apparatus which is available at the hospital for routine radiographs.

17.1.2   There is a modern 16-channel EEG machine located on Elizabeth Ward, but for some time there has been no trained technician to operate it. One of the consultant staff has had special experience and training in the field, and we recommend that urgent steps are taken to provide a technician.

17.2 Pharmacy services

17.2.1   The pharmacy services have been considerably updated in recent years. The hospital's principal pharmacist and technician are on the staff of the Nottingham Area Health Authority (Teaching) and are responsible to the Area Pharmacist. This has the advantage of providing access to the Area quality control arrangements at Nottingham as well as the drug information service of the Area Health Authority and the regional drug information service based at Leicester. A drug information bulletin is sent to all doctors at Rampton and a broad-sheet on psychiatric drugs and their potential hazard ("Psychiatric Alert") is also available.

17.2.2   Emergency drug cupboards are maintained on three wards. Statutory ward checks on drugs are carried out every three months and medicine bottles checked on return to the pharmacy every fortnight. Plans are in hand to establish a limited ward pharmacy service; we commend this development, and we hope that the additional clerical assistance required will be made available.

17.2.3   We pointed out in Chapter 13 that it is quite common practice at Rampton for drug injections to be written up 'pro re nata' (as and when required) and administered at the discretion of nursing staff. The present medicine sheets are inadequate for proper checks on this practice and modern 'Aberdeen-type' prescribing sheets should be introduced. We understand that the recently-established nursing procedures committee at the hospital is at present examining drug prescribing and administration practices with this in mind. Drug trolleys should be standard equipment on all wards.

17.2.4   The consumption of drugs can be readily checked by the excellent stock control filing system in the pharmacy. Taking into account the number of potentially restless and aggressive patients and the number of epileptics at Rampton, the overall consumption of neuroleptic and related drugs does not appear to be excessive. About half the costs of this group of drugs are accounted for by the female patients, which is in keeping with general experience—see paragraph 12.1.

17.3 Dental services

17.3.1   In considering the dental services at Rampton, we have had the benefit of the advice of our assessor, Mr G V Morrell, Area Dental Officer of Leeds Area Health Authority (Teaching) who carried out a full examination of dental facilities and examined a sample of patients and dental records.

17.3.2   Dental services are provided by a part-time general dental practitioner who has served the hospital for one year. He is assisted by a dental surgery assistant from his practice and by a staff nurse who deals with the surgery's administration.

17.3.3   The dentist attends on Wednesdays for two sessions and is available to attend for the treatment of acute cases of pain at other times. Up to 40 patients attend each day with an average attendance of 15 per session. All patients are accompanied on visits to the surgery.

17.3.4   When first appointed, the present dentist examined all the patients to assess the treatment needs, finding a high incidence of. dental disease, in many cases acute. The acute conditions were treated as a first priority and the incidence of dental emergencies has now been reduced. There were several cases in which dental disease was so advanced that removal of all the patient's teeth was the only clinical option. Most of these patients were provided with dentures, but where prostheses were not provided it was the dentist's clinical judgement that the patient would not tolerate them. Allegations have been made to us about unnecessary extraction of patients' teeth at Rampton. We wish to make it clear that our assessor's investigations found no evidence of this, and we are satisfied that if the allegations ever had any foundation (which we have no reason to believe) this is certainly not the case now. The emphasis has been on conservative dentistry. Great inroads have been made into the dental waiting list and the dentist expects to be in a position in one more year to offer routine annual inspection and treatment to all patients.

17.3.5   We were advised that the equipment in the dental surgery was obsolete and in need of replacement. We recommend that the surgery be re-equipped with modern low-seated functional equipment and that steps be taken to eliminate the noise in the surgery from compressor and aspirator motors by locating them outside. There is also a need to improve the facilities for radiographic examination including the installation of facilities for processing of plates and films.

17.3.6   Although the dentist is available to attend for the treatment of acute pain outside his normal Wednesday sessions, it appears that he is sometimes not called out in such cases and patients may have to wait for the regular surgery session, sometimes in some pain or discomfort. We recommend that a procedure for the care of dental emergencies be agreed with medical staff.

17.3.7 We think the poor state of dental health amongst patients discovered by the present dentist on his appointment points to the need for a personal oral hygiene programme operated by the nursing staff on the wards. We recommend the establishment of an in-service training programme to enable the hospital staff to undertake such a programme, which should be under the direction of the hospital dentist. To augment this preventive approach to treatment, we also recommend the appointment of a dental hygienist for two sessions per week. The catering staff need to be made fully aware of the importance of a proper diet in preventing dental disease, and of the desirability of discouraging patients so far as possible from eating snacks and sweets between meals.

17.4 Physiotherapy, speech therapy and chiropody

Three sessions weekly are provided by a physiotherapist who concentrates upon the spastic and more severely mentally handicapped patients. A chiropodist is available one day per week. We found both these services to be satisfactory. Speech therapy is not at present available, there having been no response to two advertisements. We think that speech therapy has an important role at Rampton, and hope that ways can be found of attracting interest in this post with a view to making an early appointment.

CHAPTER 18

THE NURSING STAFF

18.1 Nursing staff problems in context

18.1.1 Many of the comments which we have made in earlier chapters about various aspects of the Rampton "system" imply some criticism of the nursing staff concerned, in particular those on the male block wards. These criticisms need to be placed in their proper context. They must to a large extent be read as criticisms of the total situation within which the nurses have to work, rather than of the nurses themselves.

18.1.2 Rampton nurses at all levels must necessarily be to a large extent conditioned in their attitudes by what we have come to think of as the 'Rampton culture'. A large and geographically isolated institution like Rampton will have an innate tendency to become inward-looking, over-defensive and resistant to change. Those who are responsible for managing such an institution ought always to be on their guard against this tendency, particularly if they themselves are products of the system (see below). At Rampton however the standard of leadership provided by the medical and senior nursing staff has not in general been for the most part sufficiently positive and forward-looking to overcome 'institutional inertia'. The result has been that nursing staff have been positively discouraged by the general ethos of the hospital from adopting a critical approach to traditional attitudes and practices and trying to get changes put into effect. The situation is made worse by the fact that with a few exceptions all the nursing staff have trained at Rampton and spent all their working lives there. Many are related to one another by blood or marriage. This 'inbreeding' is largely a further product of the hospital's geographical isolation, but in addition the promotion system (see paragraph 18.4.7 below) makes it virtually impossible for nurses with substantial experience outside Rampton to be recruited at charge nurse or nursing officer level. Even at senior nursing officer level and above, only the Chief Nursing Officer (CNO) was trained outside the special hospital system.

18.1.3 Moreover, as we have already pointed out in paragraph 5.1, it is vital to bear in mind that nursing the sort of patients who find their way to Rampton can be arduous and dangerous, and that it is seldom as rewarding as nursing in other types of hospital. A number of patients have committed terrible or revolting offences before admission. It is difficult to over-estimate the amount of professional dedication and sheer hard work which the nursing staff must produce day in and day out against this background, and it is understandable that negative and over-suspicious attitudes towards patients sometimes emerge.

18.2 Nursing staff attitudes: security versus therapy

18.2.1 We discussed the question of the balance between security and therapy in general terms in paragraph 8.1–2. We think that there are a number of pressures on the Rampton nursing staff which make them tend to stress the security aspects of the work at the expense of the therapeutic. The nature of the offences which some patients have committed, the general public feeling

78

that potentially dangerous mentally disordered people should be contained in conditions of very high security, the adverse publicity which can be attracted by one disastrous failure of security, and the reluctance of many NHS hospitals to accept patients from special hospitals, all reinforce the nursing staff's perception of themselves as being primarily concerned with security. Another factor (not peculiar to Rampton) has been the steady erosion over the years of the traditional role of the psychiatric nurse by other professionals; teachers, psychologists and social workers have gradually been introduced, and now play a significant part in the patients' treatment programme, formerly carried out by nurses. This has not been seen by the nursing staff as an opportunity to enlarge and enrich their own professional nursing approach. In consequence some nursing staff see security as the one constant and measurable part of their role, and play this part at the expense of participation in patient activities being conducted by a 'specialist'. (We have seen many examples of this at Rampton). Finally, the security dilemma becomes even more complicated by the wide mix of patients on individual units. There will always be pressure to set the level of security for the ward as a whole at that appropriate for the most difficult or dangerous patient.

18.2.2   The fact that many nurses will tend, for the reasons explained above, to give priority to the security dimension of their work rather than to the therapeutic has a number of important consequences for the way the hospital is run. We have already discussed (in Chapter 11) what we think are some unacceptable aspects of the regimes on the male block wards, which stem largely from giving security an over-riding priority. A more trivial, but nonetheless instructive example is the unwillingness of some nurses to allow members of other professions—even, in some cases, doctors—to see patients by themselves, without a nurse being present to cover the security, although a shortage of suitable rooms for private interviews (see paragraphs 11.1.3 and 14.3.2) helps to justify and perpetuate this practice.

18.2.3   Too much stress on security is related to, and can easily spill over into judgmental and indeed punitive attitudes towards patients. Newly-admitted patients in particular are of course unknown quantities and a degree of caution is very necessary: there would be real dangers in forgetting why many patients have required treatment in a special hospital. However, the following extracts from reports about block ward patients show how moralistic and judgmental attitudes can at times replace a more objective account of patient behaviour: "Rather prone to argue the point, today became disgruntled when his shortcomings were highlighted. This behaviour indicates his shallow acceptance of any authority and poor self-control". "Is the definitive layabout. A still-life practitioner who can only be motivated by constant attention, he will continue to avoid work at the earliest opportunity". We do not think the attitudes revealed by comments of this sort are in general appropriate to a therapeutic environment.

18.3   Problems of nursing management

18.3.1   In the final analysis, services such as nursing are judged not on their formal structure or administrative tidiness, but on the attitudes and perceptions of individual nurses and the quality of care afforded to their patients. It is accepted however that there is a direct relationship between the quality and effectiveness of nursing management and the standards of patient care.

18.3.2 The structure of the Rampton nursing services is as follows. At the head of the nursing staff is the CNO who also has the responsibility for the School of Nursing and for security throughout the hospital. He is personally accountable to the DHSS Special Hospitals Office Committee (SHOC) (see paragraph 29.2.1). The five senior nursing officers (SNOs) of departments and areas report to him. The Principal Nursing Officer (Education) also reports to the CNO. The 16 nursing officers (NOs) who each have the responsibility for 3–4 wards, or run functional departments, report to the appropriate SNO. Charge nurses and ward sisters report to the appropriate NO.

18.3.3 The present CNO has been in post since 1974. As we pointed out previously, he is the only senior nurse manager who did not train at Rampton and he had had no previous special hospital experience before his appointment. This meant that as an 'outsider' he inevitably found himself in the front line in the battle against the institutional forces which we have described earlier. Whilst he has achieved some success in changing some time-honoured hospital practices he has allowed himself to a considerable extent to become isolated within the institution, and has not always been able to obtain the backing and support of other nurse managers when controversial decisions have had to be taken. His position has not been helped by the fact that as a member of the Hospital Executive Committee he has been required to implement decisions taken by the Policy Committee, a number of whose members are functionally subordinate to him (see paragraph 29.3.4).

18.3.4 The SNOs and NOs at Rampton wield considerable power and influence. All of them were trained (RNMS) in Rampton, and some of them have held senior positions within the POA. Several have more than one statutory qualification although their post-basic training has been almost entirely confined to management courses. As befits people who have worked their way through the ranks at Rampton they are intelligent, resourceful and perceptive, and would contribute much to any nurse management situation. It was encouraging to see some evidence of free and innovatory thinking by SNOs and NOs and concern to improve patients' standard of life.

18.3.5 It comes through clearly however that in most cases SNOs and NOs are under-extended and their potential is not being realised. In a few cases they are under-employed and do not achieve job satisfaction. Although they would be an ideal group to effect changes in attitudes and practices, they could only do so if they themselves were convinced that changes were right and necessary. At the moment, their collective views seem more sympathetic towards maintaining the traditions of the institution and towards conformity with group and institutional norms.

18.4 Our conclusions and recommendations

18.4.1 It would in our view be wholly unfair to say that nurses at any level at Rampton are in general doing their job badly. On the contrary, there is a great deal of excellent work being done at all levels. On the other hand we think that many Rampton nurses' perception of their patients' needs and their own role is, through no fault of their own, a limited and in some ways a negative one. If Rampton is to make progress, we think it is vital that those perceptions should be altered. Perceptions and attitudes can be changed only slowly and laboriously, and we are under no illusions that the recommendations we make below will produce quick or dramatic improvements. Nevertheless we are convinced that if they are adopted and given the whole-hearted backing of top management, they will eventually bear fruit.

18.4.2   We have two principal recommendations affecting the senior nursing management at Rampton both of which we think are crucial if effect is to be given to the sort of changes we have suggested above. First, we think there should be a complete review of the nursing management structure in the light of the changes we are proposing (in Chapter 29) in the management of the institution as a whole. The review would include an examination of roles, span of control and job content of the existing posts, and result in the preparation of new job descriptions for each post finally agreed. The nursing structures within the NHS will be examined as the new District Health Authorities are formed in the light of the proposals that management at 'unit' level should be strengthened and given greater financial and managerial authority. The review of nursing management at Rampton should take account of these developments. Pending the outcome of this review it is important that the executive authority of the CNO should be examined and re-stated. Management information should be available to him as of right both as a functional manager and as a member of the HMT.

18.4.3   Secondly, we think that if SNOs and NOs are to be properly equipped to lead the nursing staff in the changes of attitude which we are convinced are vital for Rampton's future, their own experience must be broadened and enlarged. A programme of visits and attachments to appropriate hospitals and outside bodies should be arranged for each officer in consultation with the Development Team for the Mentally Handicapped and the Health Advisory Service. It would be particularly valuable if countries with completely different philosophies and types of institutions could be visited.

18.4.4   We think that more junior staff too should be given every opportunity of broadening their experience and being exposed to situations which challenge and develop their existing perceptions of their role. In-service training, which we discuss in the next chapter, has a vital part to play here.

18.4.5   Although most staff are allocated to particular wards the remainder are utilised on a daily basis in a 'relief pool'. It is not uncommon for over 110 staff to be so deployed and some will have worked this way for periods in excess of a year. We are concerned at the size of this relief pool. In particular we are concerned at the way in which learner and relatively inexperienced young nursing assistants are used on relief duties. Whilst valuable experience can be gained in the pool, it may be that the length of time worked by individual nurses is overlong.

18.4.6   The style of uniform worn by the male nursing staff at NO level and below is identical to that worn by prison officers and gives what we think is an inappropriate and unhelpful symbolic expression to the custodial and non-therapeutic aspects of the nurses' role. We believe it probably reinforces many nurses' pre-occupation with those aspects of their job. We recognize that there are good security grounds for keeping a distinctive uniform of some sort for nurses, but we think that the style of the uniform should be changed to someting more appropriate to a therapeutic and caring environment.

18.4.7 We welcome the recent extablishment of a 'nursing procedures committee', which could provide Rampton with a useful forum for discussing the practical implications of changes and developments in the roles and attitudes of the nursing staff. We also welcome the introduction of the National Staff Committee (Nurses and Midwives) Staff Development and Performance Review, the principal objective of which is to improve individual performance with the ultimate objective of improving the nursing services as a whole. Within the system it is possible to identify and agree individual nurses' training and developmental needs. This would be useful in preparing programmes of visits attachments and in-service training (paragraph 18.4.3–4 above).

18.4.8 Until the early seventies, all promotion for nurses in the special hospitals up to NO level was based more or less exclusively on seniority within the hospital; only posts at SNO level and above were advertised nationally. The present system (which is the subject of a national agreement covering all special hospitals) incorporates an element of promotion on merit, but no nurse is eligible for promotion up to and including NO level unless he has served at least four years in his present grade. (In practice, this is interpreted at Rampton to mean four years *at Rampton* in his present grade). There is still no advertisement of charge nurse/ward sister or NO posts beyond Rampton and other special hospitals. In 1973 Mr Elliott recommended that all posts of charge nurse/ward sister and above should be advertised nationally (he suggested a phased introduction at charge nurse/ward sister level, with 25 per cent of vacancies advertised nationally in the first year, 50 per cent in the second year and so on) and that, to the extent that seniority should still be a factor, it must include all service and all relevant experience, wherever obtained. This recommendation had never been adopted owing, we understand, to opposition from the special hospital nursing staff. We understand that staff are concerned that an 'open' promotion system would damage the promotion prospects of staff trained at the hospital and thus cause a drain of staff away from Rampton. We are doubtful whether this would in fact be the effect of the change we are proposing. In our view the nurses' promotion system is one of the most important factors contributing to the professional isolation of the Rampton nursing staff. We are in no doubt that insofar at any rate as it applies to Rampton—we cannot make recommendations for the other special hospitals—the national agreement should be renegotiated forthwith along the lines suggested by Mr Elliott.

CHAPTER 19

THE SCHOOL OF NURSING

19.1   In considering the School of Nursing at Rampton we had the benefit of the advice of our assessor, Mr S J Holder, Director of Nurse Education at St Mary's Hospital, Paddington.

19.2   The School of Nursing is based in a modern and well-equipped staff education centre built outside the outer security perimeter. It is under the control of a Principal Nursing Officer (PNO), who is responsible to the CNO. The main role of the School is the training of student and pupil nurses for registration or enrolment with the General Nursing Council (GNC) as nurses of the mentally subnormal, although it also provides in-service training resources for the hospital as a whole (see next chapter). There are at present about 80 students and 40 pupil nurses. Our impression is that the standard of learners admitted to the School is generally high.

19.3   In addition to the PNO, the staff of the School consists of one senior tutor, two registered nurse tutors, one qualified tutor with a certificate of education, and one unqualified teacher/clinical teacher. In our view, the teaching staff are of an extremely high calibre, and compare favourably with those working in nursing schools in NHS hospitals.

19.4   The training course lasts three years for students and two years for pupils. Learners get some of their clinical experience in the wards, the industrial therapy unit and the patients' education department at Rampton, but nearly 50 per cent of their time is spent on placements in the NHS. Experience with children is obtained at Balderton Hospital, Newark and in general nursing at Victoria Hospital, Worksop. There is also a six-week community secondment.

19.5   The GNC is statutorily responsible for prescribing the standards and requirements to be met in the training of student and pupil nurses for registration and enrolment and in approving nursing schools for the purpose. The GNC periodically inspects nursing schools to ensure that these standards and requirements are being met; the last two visits to Rampton for this purpose were in 1971 and 1975. In the normal course of events a further visit would have been made in 1979. This was postponed pending completion of the police enquiries and our own work at the hospital, but we understand that it is now proposed that it should be made in the very near future.

19.6   We think that Rampton has an invaluable asset in its School of Nursing; indeed without it there would be a very large question mark hanging over the future of the hospital as a whole. If Rampton were unable to train its own nurses, it would have to attract qualified nurses who had trained elsewhere. In view of its remote geographical position and the limited appeal of the work it would, we think, find it extremely difficult to recruit sufficient qualified nurses to continue operating at all. Moreover, and equally importantly, we think that the presence of a School of Nursing is helpful in raising standards of patient care to a higher level than they would otherwise be.

19.7   Nevertheless we recognise that the School of Nursing at Rampton is facing some difficult problems and that some hard decisions are going to be necessary about the way it is to develop. The most intractable of these problems results from the change in patient mix to which we have referred in paragraph 2.4.6 and elsewhere. The number of mentally handicapped patients at Rampton is falling steadily, and is likely to continue to do so, at any rate for the next few years. The effect of this will be to limit the experience available at Rampton for mental handicap training (which is something that will clearly concern the GNC) and, conversely, make the mental handicap qualifications currently held by the majority of nurses at Rampton decreasingly relevant to the needs of the majority of the patients. At first sight the answer might appear to be to change the basic training offered at Rampton from mental handicap (RNMS for student nurses) to mental illness (RMN). But we doubt whether in the light of current developments in nurse training in both the mental illness and mental handicapped field the sort of very specialised experience which Rampton has to offer is likely for very much longer to be generally considered suitable as the main practical element in either a RNMS or RMN course.

19.8   These matters are all primarily for the GNC rather than us, and they will be able to make their own assessment of the situation when they visit the hospital. Our main point must be to stress the importance to Rampton, its patients and its staff, of ensuring that basic nurse training continues in some form or other at the hospital. But we offer a tentative suggestion which we think the GNC may wish to consider. It might be possible in the longer term for Rampton to offer training for a joint qualification in mental handicap and mental illness, but with the bulk of the practical experience obtained outside Rampton in NHS hospitals. A joint course of this sort might best be run in conjunction with an established NHS training school, preferably in a university teaching centre such as Nottingham or Sheffield. This would be an expensive option, because the prolonged placements outside Rampton would reduce the service input which the hospital gets at present from learners. But we think the price would be worth paying if it put basic nurse training at Rampton on a permanently secure footing. In addition to a joint basic course, Rampton might also provide the Joint Board for Clinical Nursing Studies' short post-qualification course on the principles of psychiatric nursing within secure environments.

19.9   We recognise that existing staff at Rampton who are registered as nurses of the mentally handicapped would be concerned that any change in the nature of basic nurse training might affect their own promotion prospects. We think the best way of meeting these fears would be by increasing in-service training and secondments orientated toward mental illness. We discuss this further in the next chapter. Some expansion of the charge nurse complement might well be necessary to meet the additional training and service demands implied by the sort of course we suggested in the previous paragraph, and this in itself would no doubt go some way towards allaying the fears of existing staff about career opportunities.

19.10   In addition to the longer-term problems discussed in the preceding paragraphs, there are some more immediate matters affecting the School of Nursing to which we think attention should be given. Many of these issues are connected with the relationship between the School and the rest of the hospital. We have found several areas where we think the balance between the educational needs of the learner and the service needs of the hospital as a whole has swung too much towards the latter. We are unhappy about the common practice whereby applicants to the School are initially recruited to the nursing assistant grade and later transferred (after a wait of up to 12 months) to an appropriate intake of learners into the School. We think this may result in learners at a time when they are at their most impressionable absorbing many of the traditional and judgmental attitudes prevalent amongst some of the longer serving nursing staff, and that these attitudes may be difficult to eradicate later. We are also concerned about the fact that when learners in the School are obtaining their practical experience in the wards and departments at Rampton, their duties are allocated, not by the School staff but by the central nursing allocations department. This often results in learners spending considerable periods doing jobs with a limited educational value such as 'escort' duties with patients attending workshops or the education department, or night duty. As part of their training programme learners are often allocated to the very large 'relief pool' of nurses which is maintained at Rampton (see paragraph 18.4.5). This means they have to work on any particular day on whatever ward has shortages, rather than being attached for a set period to a particular ward. Although the GNC has approved this practice we would prefer that as a general rule learners were attached for a set period to a particular ward. The 'long day' nursing shift system is also inappropriate for learners, for the reasons which we discussed in Chapter 10. The amount of overtime which learners work seems excessive: we heard of one student who worked 36 hours overtime in one week, and we understand it is not uncommon for learners to work on their days off.

19.11   In the light of these considerations, we have some specific suggestions to make. We think it is right that the CNO should continue to have overall responsibility for the School of Nursing and that the PNO (Education) should report him and automatically consult him over matters arising in the School with service implications. Nevertheless, we think the PNO (Education) should be operationally independent of the CNO and have complete delegated responsibility for the day-to-day running of the School. In particular, the control of the selection of students and pupils should be the responsibility of the PNO, rather than of the CNO as at present, although a representative of the service side of the hospital should always be involved in the selection process. Allocation of learners for training and secondment should be under the control of School staff. With a view to improving the quality of experience available to learners within the hospital, we think that discussions should be held to explore the possibility of identifying 'training wards', with defined objectives and with an emphasis on individual patient-care programmes. Learners should have the opportunity to attend case conferences and case reviews and the training value of these should be recognised. The hours actually spent by learners on night duty and placements outside the ward should be recorded cumulatively. The amount of overtime to be worked by learners should be agreed and should not be exceeded.

CHAPTER 20

IN-SERVICE TRAINING

20.1 Nurses' in-service training at Rampton is run by a separate in-service training section, responsible to the CNO. In-service training for other disciplines is the direct responsibility of the appropriate head of department, who has no specialist training staff to help him.

20.2 The nursing in-service training department is separate from the School of Nursing. It is run by a nursing officer, who reports to the CNO, and a charge nurse. There is no qualified teacher attached to the department: in-service training actually at the hospital is done by staff made available by the School of Nursing or by other hospital wards and departments. Secondments and outside courses are also arranged. In 1979 340 nurses were involved in training sessions, seminars or educational visits based at Rampton, mostly lasting a day or less. In the same year 38 nurses attended management courses; three nurses were seconded for RMN and one for SRN training; 11 nurses did two week secondments at hospitals for the mentally ill, and 27 staff were seconded to other authorities for courses, conferences and seminars of various kinds lasting between one day and a fortnight.

20.3 We think that Rampton needs to attach a far higher degree of importance to in-service training than it does at present. We said in the previous chapter that we think in-service training has a key role in helping nursing staff to adapt to Rampton's changing patient population. More generally, we doubt whether there is any chance at all of modifying some of the inappropriate staff attitudes we discussed in Chapter 18 without a planned programme of training and education at all levels. There should be a radical review of the education and training needs of all staff at Rampton. Management needs to be genuinely committed to the vital importance of training. It is all too easy to pay lip-service to training whilst in practice dismissing it as a distraction from one's 'real work'. There can be no place for this sort of attitude at Rampton if the hospital is to change in the ways we think it must.

20.4 The following practical steps could be taken to improve in-service training. First of all, substantially more resources must be provided. It may be that the staff complement of the School of Nursing could usefully be increased to enable the School to make a greater contribution to in-service training for nurses (and perhaps for other groups as well). But the greater part of the additional resources will in practice need to be devoted to ensuring that the staffing at all levels of the service areas of the hospital adequately reflects the fact that all staff will have to devote an increased proportion of their time to training, whether as trainers or trainees.

20.5 Secondly, there must in particular be a substantial increase in the number of nurses seconded for RMN or SRN training. We understand that the DHSS have recently authorised an increase of such secondments from four to eight a year; we welcome this as a first step and urge the hospital to ensure that the full number of secondments authorised is actually taken up. Again staffing levels must be set at a sufficient level to provide cover for nurses who are away from the hospital on secondment.

20.6   Finally, we think there is a case for organising in-service training at Rampton on a unified basis, and appointing a training officer with appropriate professional qualifications who would have the responsibility for developing and facilitating in-service training for all disciplines in the hospital. If a joint personnel department were established at the hospital (see paragraph 27.2.5) it would seem appropriate for the training officer to be attached to it. We commend this idea for further consideration by the proposed Rampton Review Board. A unified approach to training would in our view have many advantages. It would facilitate the further extension of in-service training to non-nursing groups (in particular the occupations staff whose training needs have been somewhat neglected in the past, although the position is now being remedied—see paragraph 23.5.2). It would make it easier to develop joint training sessions involving two or more disciplines, which we think have a great potential value at Rampton. Perhaps most important of all, by assigning a clear responsibility to one person within the management structure for the development of in-service training (rather than spreading the responsibility amongst a large number of senior officers as at present), it would help to ensure that training needs were given proper priority in the development of forward planning at the hospital.

CHAPTER 21

PATIENTS' ACTIVITY GROUP

21.1 There is one important function performed by nursing staff at Rampton to which we have so far alluded only briefly, and that is the organisation of what are broadly described as 'patients' activities'. Psychiatric hospitals have traditionally provided opportunities for sport and social diversion and Rampton is no exception. Since 1972 these activities have been broadened and co-ordinated by a mixed sex nursing staff team headed by a senior nursing officer and a wide range of social, sporting, occupational and training facilities have become well established. We give below some examples to show the scope of the activities provided.

21.2 Amongst the social activities organised by the Activity Group, weekly film show, discos and bingo are probably the most popular, but afternoon socials for the mentally handicapped are well attended as are the monthly concerts.

21.3 The increasing numbers of the mentally ill patients in recent years highlighted the need for an occupational activity for those male patients who were not ready, or simply unsuitable, for workshop placement. The Rehabilitative Therapy Group was formed to fulfil this need for female patients and meets each morning in the main recreation hall. Some teachers help with the development of educational and musical skills but it is mainly nurses who provide a variety of occupations which are very suitable for this type of patient.

21.4 Borderline mentally handicapped patients often attend Rehabilitative Therapy Group sessions but the needs of the highly dependent patients, male and female, are met in the mixed Play Groups. Educational rhythmics, percussion, dancing, collage and soft toy making are but a few of the wide range of pursuits which daily demonstrate the ingenuity of this very enthusiastic group of nurses. The progress being made in these two areas is of a standard which compares well with that provided in non-secure settings.

21.5 The hospital is well endowed with facilities for sporting activities and many nurses play a part in helping patients maintain and develop their skills and interests in this area. The Activity Group staff includes a charge nurse who supervises swimming and some physical education but the role of the senior activity staff is also to co-ordinate the sports run by ward-based nurses who either officiate at matches or play side by side with patients when they compete against local teams. One of the newest ventures is that of patients' mixed hockey; during the 1979/80 season Rampton has played in a local league for the first time. It has provided a valuable social experience to bring a mixed patient group together meeting a changing section of the public. (See also paragraph 31.4.2). Other more established sporting connections with the local community include football and darts while inter-ward games of table tennis, cricket and rounders are always popular. The hospital possesses two large indoor swimming pools, one of which is exclusively for patients' use. It is particularly enjoyed by sexually mixed groups of mentally handicapped patients.

21.6   There is a sports and social committee consisting of members of the staff and three patients. They make recommendations about the choice of films, social evenings and similar matters.

21.7   There is a news sheet and magazine run entirely by patients but with a member of staff as editor. A further possibility which might be considered is the provision of a hospital radio station.

21.8   The work of the Activity Group staff overlaps in several areas with that of the other rehabilitative departments which we describe in succeeding chapters. One example is the work of the Employment Bureau. This unit is run by a charge nurse, with the help of a nursing assistant or enrolled nurse, depending on availability, and it is responsible for the routine documentation and programming of patient employment and education throughout the hospital. Whenever it has been decided, for example at a case conference, that a particular patient would benefit from working in a particular workshop or from a particular class run by the patients' education department, it is the Bureau's job to match him with a vacancy.

21.9   There can be few patients who do not benefit from one or more of the many activities supervised or co-ordinated by this very adaptable group of nursing staff and we were extremely impressed by the high standard of their work.

CHAPTER 22

THE RESOCIALISATION DEPARTMENTS: GENERAL ASPECTS

22.1 The 1972 hospital policy document, to which we referred with approval in Chapter 2, said that the primary purpose of Rampton's work, apart from its security function, should be 'to prepare patients for return to the community as soon as possible'. The overall aim of Rampton is therefore essentially a rehabilitative one; as Mr Elliott said in 1973 'the whole hospital is in effect a rehabilitation department, or should be'.

22.2 As patterns of care at Rampton have evolved over the years, the roles of different groups of staff within this total rehabilitative effort have developed in different ways. A broad distinction (by no means a hard and fast one) can be drawn between medical and nursing staff on the one hand and the staff of the occupations, education, psychology and social work departments on the other. The first group have been primarily concerned with clinical aspects of the patient's total condition and, in the case of the nursing staff, with direct care of the patient, with his daily living environment and with security. The second group have been more concerned to help the patient to acquire, improve or restore the skills—educational, occupational but above all social—which he will need to function adequately outside Rampton and to relate satisfactorily to other people.

22.3 Staff in the second group are often said to be concerned with 'rehabilitation'; in view of what we said in paragraph 22.1, we think another word is required to describe the common features of their work, and agree with Mr Elliott that they are better described as 'resocialisation departments'. We do not wish to suggest however that the 'resocialisation' departments have a monopoly interest in 'resocialisation': a large part of the work of doctors and nurses at Rampton, or indeed in any psychiatric hospital, will be concerned with 'resocialisation' in the widest sense of the word.

22.4 Mr Elliott said that the occupations, education, psychology and social work departments formed a kind of 'resocialisation group'. 'They ought to work together as one group' he said. 'The psychology department ought to be directly involved in defining the policies of the occupations department, whose activities, together with education, farm, library, playgroups and so on, ought to be seen as a joint venture, aiming at well thought out objectives, and linking in with the work of doctors and nurses at every level and at every turn'. We agree wholeheartedly with this as an objective for the resocialisation departments. We have not found however that very much progress has been made towards achieving this objective since Mr Elliott reported in 1973. There have been few attempts to co-ordinate the programme offered by the different resocialisation departments, although in fairness it must be pointed out that staff shortages, particularly in the psychology and social work departments, have made such attempts much more difficult. Similarly liaison between the resocialisation departments and medical and nursing staff has often been poor (although good relations have been built up between the nurses' Activity

Group, whose work we described in the previous chapter, and the occupations and education departments). Inter-professional rivalries have certainly contributed to poor liaison; as we pointed in paragraph 18.2.1, the nursing staff in particular must often feel to some extent threatened by the apparent erosion of their role by resocialisation group staff, whereas in fact their work is complementary and overlapping.

22.5   We agree with Mr Elliott that the work of the patients' library should be regarded as closely allied to that of the resocialisation departments. We take the opportunity of commending the excellent service provided by the patients' library at Rampton, including the toy library provided for mentally handicapped patients.

22.6   We think that every opportunity should be taken of increasing mutual understanding and co-operation both between the individual resocialisation departments and between them and the rest of the hospital. Joint in-service training of the kind we suggested in Chapter 20 would make an important contribution to this, but we think that some formal administrative machinery is also necessary. We were pleased to learn that since we have been working at Rampton a committee has been set up, with members from all disciplines, 'to review the need for increasing communication and co-ordination between those disciplines involved in treatment and rehabilitation, to review the current facilities available to the patient and to report as to their appropriateness to the patient's rehabilitation'. In our proposals for a revised management structure, we recommend (paragraph 29.4.5) that there should be a resocialisation team, comprising the heads of the education, psychology, occupations and social work departments, the SNO (Activities) and a doctor nominated by the Medical Advisory Committee. The librarian might also attend when necessary. The team's principal function would be to plan and co-ordinate the services offered by the resocialisation departments to the clinical teams. We hope this will help quicker progress towards making resocialisation programmes at Rampton the 'joint venture' which Mr Elliott envisaged.

CHAPTER 23

THE OCCUPATIONS DEPARTMENT

23.1 The department and its staff

23.1.1 The aims of the occupations department as stated in its recently produced 'policy and strategy statement' (see paragraph 29.7) are to provide therapeutic occupational activities for patients, which supplement the other specialist treatments they receive, and which are designed to assist each patient's rehabilitation by developing regular work habits and creative interests, by teaching basic social and manual skills, and by giving support and encouragement in a secure working environment. These activities are provided in 28 male workshops, in an Industrial Training Unit (ITU), and on the female verandahs (see 23.3.1), and also in other areas of the hospital (laundry, kitchen, etc) or its grounds. About 400 male and 100 female patients—about five-eighths of the total patient population—attend occupations activities during 'working hours'—roughly 9.00–12.00 and 13.00–16.45 Monday to Friday. Most workshops carry out work for the hospital itself and also for staff, patients' relatives and the public, which earns a substantial income (about £29,000 in 1979/80) for the hospital.

23.1.2 The department is staffed by 'occupations staff', a group peculiar to the special hospitals. Some are ex-nurses who have appropriate skills; others are craftsmen who have been recruited direct. Their pay is linked to various nursing grades. The Department is headed by a Chief Occupations Officer who is directly responsible to the hospital managers (DHSS). At the time of writing he is supported by five senior occupations officers, 35 occupations officers and 42 occupations assistants. It has been accepted however that these numbers are insufficient to provide adequate cover for sickness, holidays, attendance at case conferences and in-service training, and an increase of 25 in the complement (bringing the total to 108) has recently been authorised.

23.1.3 Occupations staff are responsible not only for teaching patients basic job skills and supervising and assessing their work, but also for escorting them to and from the workshops and for security in the workshops, where tools and materials present a considerable risk. They are the only non-nursing staff in the hospital who take sole responsibility for the security of individual patients.

23.1.4 Patients' performance at work is encouraged by a 'points' system. Patients can earn points by performing satisfactorily at work, up to a maximum which is fixed separately for each workshop depending on the level of work done. Points earned are converted into a nominal monetary sum which is credited to the patient and which he can either spend (in the hospital shop or using mail order), remit to his family or save. The system has been operating more or less unchanged for a number of years. It requires a radical overhaul and we are pleased to learn that it is currently being examined by a working party at the hospital.

23.1.5   The workshops are scattered over a wide area and the long-term objective is to re-locate them in one area. Many of the shops have inadequate facilities; some lack toilets (which poses security problems in addition to the problems of hygiene); some are inadequately heated; and there is a general lack of storage space. Management is aware of these shortcomings which are being gradually remedied as financial and other restraints permit.

23.2   The male workshops

23.2.1   Following his initial assessment period (see Chapter 9.3) a male patient who is considered suitable for occupational activity will normally be assigned to one of the 28 workshops, covering a wide range of trades and crafts*, to the patients' kitchen, or to the ITU. The ITU is for the less able patients, and carries out mainly light industrial work of a repetitive nature such as assembling toys. During 1979 there was a marked reduction in orders obtained for the ITU and this caused some concern. However, the appointment of a new full-time Industrial Liaison Officer has already resulted in a noticeable increase in the amount and variety of new work.

23.2.2   There are occupational activities for men in other areas, but these are not usually made available until the patient has made a certain amount of progress through the 'system'. These are the printing shop (which is 'integrated' with female patients attending as well), the hospital stores, and for pre-discharge patients, the working parties which operate outside the secure area—farm and gardens and pig farm (also integrated) and concrete construction. We think that the work being done in the farms and gardens and pig farm fulfils a particularly valuable rehabilitative function.

23.2.3   When new patients arrive in the workshops or the ITU they are usually interviewed by the occupations officer in charge and after simple routine tasks to test their ability are placed on suitable work. Progress is carefully monitored and work changed according to the patients' needs. Basic skills are taught with great success and for this the occupations officers deserve full credit. There is a good working relationship with patients; the atmosphere in the workshops is pleasant and relaxed and there are relatively few disturbances or violent incidents.

23.3   The female workshops

23.3.1   The new female patients will normally be allocated either to the sewing room (which repairs all hospital clothing and is under the control of the Administrator's department) or to one of the 'verandah workrooms'. A variety of activities are carried on in these workrooms—diversional therapy, repetitive industrial tasks and simple food preparation for the least able patients, and handicrafts and light industrial tasks of various sorts for the rest.

23.3.2   Later on female patients may have the opportunity of working in the (integrated) printing shop, the staff kitchen, the laundry or an integrated outside party working in the gardens.

---

*Shoemaking, tailoring, metalwork, brushmaking, carpentry, baking, upholstery, weaving, toymaking, traditional handcrafts, bookbinding, basketwork, pottery, concrete slab manufacture.

23.4 Our assessment of the department's work

23.4.1 In general, we were impressed by the work of the occupations department. In 1972 Mr Elliott found it unsure of its role and lacking in adequate leadership. Since then it has made considerable progress under the competent leadership of the present Chief Occupations Officer. The patients clearly enjoy participating in the department's activities as the relaxed atmosphere in the workshops testifies, and we think those activities make an extremely useful contribution to the overall rehabilitative effort of the hospital. We think nevertheless there are some areas in which further progress could and should be made.

23.4.2 There are in our view two areas in particular where the choice of occupational activity on offer is insufficient to meet patients' needs. Firstly we think it ought to be possible to provide the more able female patients with rather more intensive and challenging activities than at present, both initially and as they progress towards discharge or transfer. Secondly we think that for both male and female pre-discharge patients there should be a wider range of activities available in low security conditions. As we indicated in paragraph 23.2.2 above, when patients have progressed to a villa and their transfer or release from Rampton appears likely, they are normally transferred to an outside working party to test their reaction to less secure conditions. The only options offered are gardening and concrete construction work; there is a lack of sufficient industrial-type work options to test a patient's suitability for discharge or transfer, and prepare him for it, under near normal conditions (including a working day of a realistic length) and an unobtrusive security regime. We understand that in order to remedy this it has been agreed by the hospitals' Policy Committee that a workshop should be set up in a building within the hospital grounds but just outside the outer security fence. Little progress in implementing this decision has however been made largely, we understand, because of difficulty in obtaining the agreement of the POA. We believe that this project must go ahead if patients are to be helped to learn normal patterns of working behaviour, are to be properly assessed under as near as possible to normal 'outside' conditions and are to be fully prepared to leave Rampton. In general we think that the options for work available to pre-discharged patients should so far as possible be orientated towards preparing them for the sort of work they might reasonably expect to take up on discharge.

23.4.3 We drew attention earlier in Chapter 7 to the therapeutic benefits we feel could be derived from a careful extension of integration of the sexes among patients, and suggested that some of the workshops might be good places to start. There is already integration in the printing shop, and the garden working party. We understand that the Industrial Liaison Officer and the new rehabilitation committee (see paragraph 22.6) are considering how further integration can be achieved; we suggest that integration could be tried first on the (female) verandah workrooms and in the (male) pottery workshops.

23.4.4 As we indicated in Chapter 22, we found a tendency at Rampton to treat the trade training programme (like the other resocialisation pro-

94

grammes) as an end in itself, rather than linking it with the medical and nursing needs of the patient. Liaison between occupations staff and medical and nursing staff leaves much to be desired. The occupations officers return patients to the wards early on Tuesday afternoons in order to have time for ward discussion with nurses, but whilst this is welcomed it coincides with a busy time on the ward and if several occupations officers wish to speak to the same charge nurse/ward sister the difficulties are intensified. Many charge nurses/ward sisters fail to let occupations officers know of changes in the patient's medication which might affect workshop performance. Consultants appear to visit the workshops rarely if at all so they rely entirely upon other people's reports when assessing a patient's suitability for a particular task and monitoring his reactions to it thereafter. Closer links must be established between doctors, nurses and the occupations department in the interests of better therapeutic care for the patient.

23.5 Occupations staff problems

23.5.1 Appointments to the occupations department are usually made at occupations assistant level but the salary scale (which is the same as that of a nursing assistant) is not attractive to outside craftsmen. Staff cannot transfer from nursing without a considerable drop in pay owing to the loss of overtime and unsocial hours payments; this is a serious drawback as in the past many occupations officers had a nursing background which was useful in their daily work and helpful in nurse/occupations officer relationships. Because of low staff turnover at occupations officer level, opportunities for promotion are relatively rare; it is therefore difficult to provide an attractive career structure for occupations assistants. While recruitment at occupations assistant level is possible under the present local economic situation there is little doubt that many occupations assistants would leave Rampton once trades positions became available outside. We feel that the DHSS should as a matter of urgency take steps to provide a career structure and realistic pay scale for occupations assistants. We recognise of course that any implications for the principle of linkage between nurses and occupations staff pay will need to be taken into account. One possibility might be to provide a number of posts at occupations officer level which could be held supernumerary to establishment and allocated by the head of department to occupations assistants who satisfied certain defined and agreed criteria. We are in no doubt that the whole department has a feeling of deep injustice over pay and conditions of service and this should be faced as soon as possible.

23.5.2 Little formal training takes place for occupations staff, but efforts are being made to improve this. There is a two-week combined course for occupations assistants and nursing assistants which has been attended by most occupations assistants. A draft course has been prepared for occupations officers under which they will undergo a day's training once a week for nine weeks, followed by four weeks working on the wards for three days each week. As this course is being prepared jointly with the Chief Nursing Officer it should both help occupations officers in their normal duties and also make a useful contribution to nurse/occupations officer relationships.

CHAPTER 24

THE EDUCATION DEPARTMENT

24.1 In considering the education department at Rampton we had the benefit of the advice of our assessor, Mr C A Norman, formerly Her Majesty's Inspector (Staff Inspector) at the Department of Education and Science.

24.2 The department and its staff

24.2.1 The education department sees its duties as twofold: to make available to patients the type of educational provision that would normally be available to them if they were living in the community, ie adult education; and to provide an educational programme which will assist the hospital to meet its aims of preparing patients for return to the community as soon as possible.

24.2.2 The department has gone on to identify four major functions which it must perform in order to discharge these duties.

a. The development in patients of a higher level of social competence through the improvement of basic communication skills. Four types of course are offered to meet this objective:

i. a programme of activities for severely mentally handicapped patients to develop perceptual and physical skills, and assist concentration, motivation and the use of language;

ii. a remedial programme for illiterate and semi-illiterate patients designed to improve communication skills;

iii. a basic studies course for educationally backward patients seeking to improve basic education skills and to apply them in everyday social situations; and

iv. a course on self-care skills—including basic cooking, washing and ironing, repair of clothing and household budgeting—for male pre-discharge patients.

b. The provision of opportunity for more able patients to further their academic development. Classes are provided in English and mathematics up to 'O' level standard. Other subjects may be studied by correspondence course. A few patients have followed Open University courses financed from hospital funds.

c. To widen the patients' range of general interests. Classes of a recreational and non-vocational nature, each of two hours a week, are available mainly in the evenings.

d. To provide vocational education. At present this is restricted to a one-year part-time course on 'basic cooking for the catering industry' and a typewriting course.

24.2.3 The staff of the department are employed by the Nottinghamshire Local Education Authority who meet all the day-to-day running costs (mostly refunded to them by DHSS). Heading the department is a Senior Education Officer who is responsible jointly to the local authority's Director of Education and to DHSS as managers of the hospital. The teaching staff consists of a deputy head, nine full-time teachers (two of them are new posts added in January 1980), four part-time teachers working during the day and about a dozen part-time staff employed for evening classes. A staff nurse is seconded to the department and is responsible for the internal movement of patients to and from classes and for overall security while patients are in the department. Education is provided by the teachers for approximately 43 weeks in the year: teachers receive holidays of the normal length but these are staggered to avoid any closure for more than three weeks during the year.

24.2.4 Over 400 patients receive education during term-time, each for an average of just over five hours a week. Most classes are co-educational. Most teaching is done in the education centre, a single storey building in the inner secure area which used to be a weaving shed. It is rather cramped, and additional accommodation has recently been brought into use. The education department is adequately furnished and is well provided with audiovisual aids, including television, a video recorder and a number of small teaching machines. The department is also responsible for the hospital gymnasium, and has the use of the recreation hall and the patients' swimming pool at certain times. Some education work is also done on the wards. Education staff assist Activity Group nursing staff in running Rehabilitative Therapy groups (see paragraph 21.3) and are also involved in social advisory groups for pre-discharge patients.

24.3 Our assessment of the department's work

24.3.1 Few other educational institutions are concerned with students who have such a wide range of ability and personality problems and the teachers at Rampton are faced with a most exacting task. The staff are particularly well equipped to meet this challenge; the Senior Education Officer provides good leadership and the department's work is deservedly well respected in the hospital. The education staff show a deep commitment to their work which manifests itself in their attitude to the students. All the classes we observed had been thoroughly prepared by the teachers who were always courteous and encouraging towards their students. As a result, relationships between teachers and students are remarkably good and the atmosphere in classes was relaxed, yet without any loss of effort or application on the part of the students.

24.3.2 There is however one serious organisational problem which to a very substantial extent frustrates all this good work by the teachers and which must be mentioned at this stage. This is the problem of lack of punctuality by patients. Patients who attend classes are escorted to and from their sessions by members of the nursing staff. Because of nurses' ward duties, and delays in the afternoon caused by the meal rotas, we found that patients regularly arrived up to 30 minutes late and not uncommonly 45 minutes to an hour late. This can occur at the beginning of any of the three sessions, morning, afternoon or evening. For similar reasons, patients are also often taken away early from classes. This unpunctuality results in a serious waste of resources since teachers are being paid for the time that is lost. It causes frustration to the teaching staff as well as impairing the efficiency of the education programme. The problem should be given urgent attention. Changes in the nursing shift system (see Chapter 10) could partly alleviate it by reducing the disruption caused by nursing staff meal breaks. Such changes might also make it possible for patients attending classes to enjoy the one hour's exercise at lunch time, which occupations patients have, instead of being confined to the wards for this period. Another solution might be to have particular nurses attached to the education department to escort patients to class and to provide security supervision while they are there. If nurses with a specific interest in education were chosen for this duty, they could assist with the teaching programmes; at present many nurses merely sit watching and are patently not involved.

24.3.3   So far as the work of the education department itself is concerned, our observation and examination identified areas however where we think the level (rather than the quality) of service could be enhanced. We fully realise that any extension of provision will have staff or other resource implications and will require detailed consideration locally to determine the most efficient way of achieving it. In the rest of this chapter we have therefore restricted ourselves to identifying the areas in which we think change or development is desirable and making some tentative suggestions. We look to the proposed new resocialisation team (see paragraph 22.6) to consider and develop our suggestions further.

24.4   Areas for development

24.4.1   We are sure that more patients than at present could benefit from the education services—at present about half do not. In November 1979, at the time when we were doing our field work at the hospital, there were substantial waiting lists for education—83 for day classes and 54 for evening classes. Even so, demand has no doubt to a large extent adjusted itself to supply, and if more facilities were available a different view would almost certainly be taken of many patients who are not at present considered suitable for education. We think that money spent on expanding the educational facilities at Rampton would certainly be money well spent. Most of the actual financial cost would fall on DHSS, as explained in paragraph 24.2.3 above, but we hope that the local education authority would co-operate by approving any necessary increases in complement. Perhaps the first step in developing services might be to put in hand a special survey of the patient population to estimate how many might benefit from various given levels of additional provision.

24.4.2   In particular, we would like to see the further (ie adult) education programme widened and developed. For patients who are long-stay residents in hospital, recreational activities are much more significant, even crucial, than for the normal clients of further education provision. A comprehensive programme can not only help individuals in their development and rehabilitation; it can also make the day-by-day- management of patients much easier for staff on duty. At present, further education is mainly restricted to two evenings in the week. The known demand for classes from the patients may not be a reliable guide to what is needed unless patients can be made fully aware of the implications and possibilities of a fuller further education programme and the range of classes that can be made available.

24.4.3   The opportunities for vocational training should also be extended;

at present, as indicated above, they are limited to courses in cookery and typing. Any further vocational courses could very usefully be co-ordinated with the provisions for training that are currently available in the occupations workshops.

24.4.4　We think that the day-time courses could be further developed with courses for example in social and environmental studies, language, literature and art and craft. This would help meet the needs of the more able patients for whom provision is at present limited.

24.4.5　The fact that most education classes are co-educational adds to their overall usefulness considerably. We think there may be scope for building on this and developing integrated social skills and sex education courses for a wider range of patients in conjunction with the clinical psychology department.

24.4.6　Teachers do undertake some work with groups and individuals on wards. At present five groups of patients are involved, most for two hours a week, and a few patients are given individual tuition in shorter sessions. We suggest that a thorough re-appraisal should be undertaken of the needs in all wards. This appraisal is only likely to be effective if the multidisciplinary clinical teams are fully aware of the part education can play in programmes for the management and treatment of patients whose behaviour problems are both complex and serious.

24.4.7　A number of cases of severely and profoundly deaf students were brought to our notice. All but one of these are men under 30 years of age. The teaching staff try to give special teaching to these patients but, so far as we know, none of them has been assessed by a specialist teacher of the deaf. We think that specialist assessment and guidance, including the services of an audiologist, can be crucial for these patients and that it should be available on a regular basis to the education department. It would also help if a sign language course was run for a small group of nursing staff who look after these patients.

24.4.8　We think that patients should be given better guidance on the options for study open to them if they are to take full advantage of the opportunities available. It is important that those of low ability and limited educational achievement who may have been discouraged by past educational failures should be helped to understand as fully as possible what the various courses can offer. Patients appear to be heavily dependent on the advice of the nurses on their wards when selecting courses; in some cases nurses are well informed and able to help but this is not always so. Further thought should be given to ways of assisting patients in making their choices.

24.4.9　There is a need for strengthening links between the education department and the nursing and occupations staff. All professional groups are represented at case conferences and this contact is of course helpful in extending understanding between the disciplines. We would however like to see teachers taking every opportunity to visit the wards to discuss patients' needs and progress with the nurses, and vice versa. We found the system of attaching nurses to the education centre for a time as part of their initial training to be particularly useful. We would also like to see the introduction of integrated programmes for patients devised jointly by the occupations and education staff (see for example 24.4.3 above). The proposed resocialisation team should provide a forum in which these ideas can be developed.

24.4.10   Links between the education department and educational organisations outside the hospital are very limited. The teaching staff work in a situation of considerable professional isolation. There are occasional links with further education colleges in the area, usually over specialist courses, and some staff have contacts with universities and colleges in connexion with the in-service studies they undertake. Contacts with local education authority advisers are infrequent. The isolation reflects the undoubted difficulty there is in finding outside contacts which are likely to be helpful. Perhaps the educational provision that has most in common with that at Rampton is that provided in prisons. The Home Office Prisons Education Service makes regional arrangements for meetings of staff and for in-service training and we think it would be helpful if the teachers at Rampton were able to make and maintain contact with this service and take advantage of any training and advisory services that were available.

24.4.11   We pointed out in paragraph 24.2.3 that the staff of the department are employed by Nottinghamshire Local Education Authority although most of the costs are refunded to them by DHSS. This agency type of arrangement has had advantages in the past. At a time of restriction of local authority expenditure there is nevertheless a danger that the education authority may seek to restrict development at Rampton on principle or for uniformity even though costs incurred will be fully reimbursed. Should such a conflict occur, we think it may be necessary to consider direct employment of the education staff.

CHAPTER 25

THE CLINICAL PSYCHOLOGY DEPARTMENT

25.1 We find it difficult to adopt the same format in this chapter as we have adopted in the two immediately preceding ones, first of all giving a description of the objectives of the department, its staff and working methods, then going on to give an assessment of its work and suggest areas for improvement. This is because during the period we were working at Rampton the clinical psychology department nearly ceased to exist at all.

25.2 At the time we started work at Rampton the official establishment of clinical psychologists at Rampton was five—a Principal Clinical Psychologist as head of the department, two senior clinical psychologists and two basic grade or probationer clinical psychologists. Only two of these posts were actually filled, the Principal and one senior. During the course of our work, the Principal resigned to take up an appointment in the NHS. This left the senior to run the department single-handed. The Principal vacancy was advertised, but no suitable candidate applied. At this stage we advised the DHSS that in our view the importance of clinical psychology at Rampton was such that the department should be headed by a Top Grade Clinical Psychologist. The DHSS agreed with this recommendation and at the time of writing a Top Grade Post (which will be in addition to rather than a substitute for the Principal post) has been advertised. Meanwhile the department continued to be run by only one psychologist, (although we now understand that a probationer has recently been appointed).

25.3 We have already made it clear in a number of places in our report how important we consider the role of clinical psychologists at Rampton. There are a large number of patients at the hospital, including many of those with sexual problems and many mentally handicapped patients with propensities towards violence or other forms of deviant behaviour, to whom psychological techniques offer the best hope of any real improvement in their condition. There must be adequate psychological input into the assessment procedures (paragraph 9.3.3) but, more importantly, there is little hope of introducing flexibility into treatment regimes and developing individual behaviour modification, self-care and social skills programmes (paragraph 7.3.3) unless there are psychologists fully involved in the work of the clinical teams. They must be able to design suitable programmes and train other staff, particularly nurses, actually to operate them in the wards and departments. Clinical psychologists could play an important role in psychotherapy, both on an individual and a group basis. They could make useful contributions to the work of the resocialisation departments as a whole; the 'points' system (paragraph 23.1.4) was originally designed by a clinical psychologist. The appointment of more clinical psychologists would provide some welcome support for the medical staff (paragraph 16.2.6).

25.4 We shall not attempt to assess the past work of the psychology department at Rampton in the light of the functions which we have suggested for it in the previous paragraph. All that we really need to say is that during most of the period of our work, despite valiant efforts by the solitary member of the department in post during that time, its input to Rampton as a whole was insignificant. We hope that the new head of the department will be able to take a completely fresh look at its role, and discuss with his professional colleagues in other disciplines at the hospital the best way in which in practice, in the light of staff resources available, that role can be discharged. But the first priority must clearly be to ensure that the Department is adequately staffed.

25.5   There is a national shortage of clinical psychologists which means that qualified people have a wide choice of jobs. Rampton's isolation is clearly an important factor in deterring psychologists from applying for posts at Rampton, but it is not the only one; no other department at Rampton has had anything like the same difficulties in attracting staff. The accommodation hitherto used by the department is most unsatisfactory, being leaky, cramped and badly laid out, and this may have put off some potential applicants. A new building has now been authorised; we understand that work should begin in 1980 and this may go some way toward helping recruitment. But we suggest there may in the past have been other rather less tangible reasons why psychologists have found the prospect of working at Rampton less than inviting. These may well have had a great deal to do with the perceptions both of previous heads of the department and of the other professional groups at Rampton of what the role and status of the clinical psychologist at Rampton should be. As we have made clear, our firm view is that clinical psychologists are absolutely vital to the future of Rampton. We think that this must be recognised by the management of the hospital and by all the staff (particularly doctors and nurses) if the department is to have any chance of successfully 'selling' itself to potential recruits. The Medical Director (see paragraph 16.7.6–7 and Chapter 29) will have an important part to play in bringing this about.

25.6   Another way we think it might be possible to make Rampton a more attractive place to clinical psychologists is by developing research and teaching links with universities. Consideration could be given to joint appointments with universities or to securing honorary University status for Rampton staff. This is something which the new head of the department should be asked to explore urgently.

25.7   We think the establishment of the department should be increased above its present levels. In addition to the Top Grade Clinical Psychologist there should be two Principal Psychologists (each attached to one of the two male clinical teams), a senior clinical psychologist (attached to the female team), two basic grade and two probationer psychologists. One of the two basic grade psychologists should be a specialist in work with the mentally handicapped; we think in the past the department may have concentrated a little too many of its scarce resources on work with the more able mentally ill patients. There was a male staff nurse permanently attached to the department but this post has recently been withdrawn. The male nurse undertook security and escort duties and also some assessment and therapeutic work. We recommend that this post should be restored and, in addition, a female staff nurse should also be appointed. Her functions would be to develop social training for male patients and also, by undertaking escort and security duties, to enable female patients to be seen in the department. A technician should be appointed as soon as possible (there is a vacancy at present), and adequate secretarial and clerical help should be made available.

CHAPTER 26

THE SOCIAL WORK DEPARTMENT

26.1 The department and its staff

26.1.1 The social work department sees its role as 'to facilitate, in co-operation with the patients, families, other hospital disciplines and community services, the effective rehabilitation of men and women detained in Rampton back into normal community life'.

26.1.2 The department is housed temporarily (although probably for some years yet) in a pleasant building, previously an estate house, outside the secure area. There would be advantages if the social work staff were based nearer to colleagues in other disciplines but we are told that this is not practicable within available accommodation. Social workers visit the block wards, villas and other sections of the hospital to see patients and staff. One advantage of being outside the secure area is the easy access it gives for patients' visitors and community contacts such as legal representatives and probation officers.

26.1.3 The present establishment consists of one Principal Social Worker, one deputy, and ten social workers (all paid on social worker level 3 grade scales on the basis that it is essential that they should all have had previous experience). The Principal Social Worker is directly responsible to the hospital managers (DHSS). When we began work at the hospital, there had been three or four vacancies for several months, and although all but one were taken up, the section now again has three vacancies. There are however several applicants for these posts. One further post has been agreed in principle by the Policy Committee but not yet advertised. There is also one clerical officer and one clerical assistant attached to the department. The Principal has done well in establishing the work of the department on such a firm basis since it was set up in its present form in 1973.

26.1.4 The professional standards of the staff are good. The contribution they can make to the well-being of patients through multidisciplinary work and management is now established although it must be said that some consultants are less enthusiastic than others as regards multidisciplinary planning. There are still some nursing staff who have difficulty in accepting the role of social workers (particularly the counselling role described in paragraph 26.3 below) but we believe the majority acknowledge the contribution which they can make to the present and future care of patients and their families. This tension between groups of staff is not peculiar to Rampton; it can arise in any institution where one group see themselves as carrying the brunt of patients' care and regard other groups as outsiders. It can become a serious problem if allowed to develop and its avoidance must be consciously worked at by all parties. What we said in Chapter 22 about relations between the resocialisation departments and the rest of the hospital is of course of direct relevance to this problem.

26.1.5 In their work with patients and their families, the tasks of the social work staff can be broadly split into three distinct areas: initial assessment and contact with a patient's family; counselling and other work on the wards; and pre-discharge work. These are discussed separately below.

26.2 Initial assessment and family contact

As part of the initial assessment of a new patient a home visit is generally done, where any home exists. We were told that relatives welcome these visits and they are therefore regarded not only as part of case history taking but also as a public relations exercise for Rampton. Social workers attempt to combine two or three visits to the same area, but this is not always possible because of Rampton's nationwide catchment area. Consequently, they have to spend a considerable proportion of their time travelling, which reduces their effectiveness. Local authority and probation workers often undertake subsequent visits to a patient's home but they are at a disadvantage as they rarely know the patient personally. Some patients who have been at Rampton a long time have not had a home visit and their records therefore lack or are inadequate in personal histories.

26.3 Counselling and ward work

Counselling of various kinds is undertaken by staff from every discipline including the social workers. Given sufficient staff we would hope to see an increase in the social work contribution in selected cases. There is room for participation in group discussions of a therapeutic nature, which would provide a valuable additional element for inclusion in treatment programmes. Psychologists and social workers worked together in groups in the past but progress had stopped because of the staffing problems in both departments. Co-operation with the education department and nursing staff, particularly on the pre-discharge villas, has also been fruitful. We hope that social workers will be able to resume their involvement in group discussions, and that some of them will be given the opportunity of further training in this field. We understand that as social work staff have been appointed some groups have now in fact been restarted.

26.4 Pre-discharge work

26.4.1 As we described in Chapter 15, patients are discharged from Rampton to their homes, hostels or lodgings or are transferred to other hospitals. The social work department has an important role at this stage of the patient's career, and often faces a number of problems, not the least being to convey to the receiving authority and hospital staff that the patient is ready and able to function in the community with limited supervision. Because of the difficulties in finding as well as funding placements to which we referred in paragraph 15.7, the social workers find themselves involved in exploring a number of alternatives, often at an early stage when it is difficult to give a firm view of the patient's likely behaviour in a non-secure setting. Some receiving hospitals insist on having the local authority's assurance that they will bear the financial responsibilities of the patient's eventual discharge, but few local authorities are willing to give this in advance for a variety of reasons, not the least being a shortage of funds. Additional problems for social workers can arise when discharges occur without adequate notice, for example when MHRTs make a decision to discharge. Most authorities are willing to undertake supervision on discharge of a patient but Rampton's social workers often have difficulty in locating the right contact within a large local authority. Updating local information on hostels and lodgings, and the personalities and abilities of their staff is also very important, if the placement is to be successful, and together with the arrangements for financial support of discharged patients takes a great deal of social workers' time. We recommend in paragraph 15.7 that the DHSS should extend the present very limited facilities for giving financial assistance to enable patients to be supported in specialist hostels.

26.4.2 Some time ago the Principal Social Worker planned with a co-operative local authority in the Midlands to place one of the Rampton social workers part-time in the area. The local authority agreed to provide office space and clerical support. The area was chosen because of the number of patients coming from surrounding districts. Broadly, the intention was that the Rampton social worker would spend perhaps about a quarter of his time based in the area, improving contacts with local authorities, hospitals and voluntary agencies, obtaining up to date information on local facilities, giving support to local social workers over patients in hostels in the community, and visiting families where appropriate. The experiment could not be pursued because of shortage of social workers at Rampton. Now the staff position has improved, we think it would be worth reviving.

26.5 Staff matters

26.5.1 One suggestion that has been put to us is that Rampton social workers should be employed by the local authority (like the teachers in the Rampton education department and social workers working in NHS hospitals) rather than by DHSS. We can see some attractions in this idea, particularly if it provided social workers at Rampton with more accessible professional support and advice than under the present arrangements, and would not wish to rule it out altogether if it were what the staff themselves wanted. We are not however convinced that the case for change is sufficiently clear for us to make a definite recommendation. The position would certainly need to be looked at if Rampton's catchment area were ever 'regionalised' (see paragraphs 4.1–2).

26.5.2 Social workers' salaries and grading are based on those of local authority social services department staff, but their other terms and conditions of service are based on those of NHS hospital social workers before the transfer to local government employment in 1974, subsequently amended from time to time. Rampton social workers during the period of our review did not appear to have a clear idea of their terms and conditions of service: the DHSS, at our suggestion, have produced a consolidated statement and made it available to all staff.

26.5.3 Because until recently the department has been substantially below complement, it has been difficult to estimate accurately whether the existing complement is adequate for the amount of work and whether the grade structure within the department is right. The staffing position has now improved and we think there should be a review of staffing levels in one year's time, by which time the department should have had sufficient experience of running on more or less full complement. Meanwhile, we think that the additional post that has been agreed in principle should be advertised forthwith and that this post should be raised to the level of second deputy. The incumbent could undertake special duties such as work with local authorities and voluntary bodies to encourage support for patients and relatives, and also in the field of discharge such as securing the provision of accommodation.

26.5.4   Opportunities for social workers to attend full-time further training and short courses needs to be maintained and expanded. There should be provision for the regular exchange of ideas and information with staff at the other special hospitals. Additional training provision should help to improve standards and provide an attraction in recruiting staff. Joint training with staff from other disciplines within the hospital might help in establishing better understanding of each other's contributions towards the well-being of patients (see Chapter 20).

26.5.5   Social workers have to spend a lot of time on routine duties such as tracking down patients' relatives for record purposes and dealing with queries about patients' credit-worthiness from mail order companies. Steps should be taken to relieve social workers of duties of this sort, perhaps by increasing the level of clerical support.

CHAPTER 27

THE ADMINISTRATOR AND HIS DEPARTMENT

27.1 General considerations

27.1.1   The role of the hospital Administrator is in essence the same in a special hospital as in any other psychiatric hospital. The Administrator and his staff are responsible for the domestic institutional and support services (see Chapter 28) and are the principal guides and interpreters of the general management systems. They play no direct part in the treatment of patients but since they provide the milieu in which doctors and nurses work and patients live, their contribution is important. The caring professions may know the changes and developments they would like to see introduced to improve the hospital and its services but they rely heavily on the Administrator's knowledge of the general management systems and his ability to interpret and deploy them effectively to translate plans into reality. Another important aspect of the Administrator's work is to act as the principal channel of communication with the public; he is apart from the day-to-day care of patients and is thus well qualified to direct the investigation of complaints and to supervise the proper administration of the Mental Health Act as it affects Rampton patients. He also has an important role to play in consultations with staff and industrial relations.

27.1.2   Although the special hospitals are not part of the NHS they are heavily influenced by it and this is particularly apparent in management and administrative arrangements. However, their separation is valuable to the extent that it enables them to be selective in adopting particular aspects of NHS management practice.

27.1.3   The current criticism of the NHS, that managment at hospital level has been emasculated, is not true of the Administrator's department at Rampton. In this regard Rampton is a good example of a local 'unit' of management which the current NHS reorganisation is designed to restore; indeed since more functions are managed directly by the Administrator in a special hospital than in a NHS hospital, notably finance and supplies, Rampton in this respect goes beyond anything the NHS currently aims to achieve. There are many aspects of administration where the special hospitals are in a privileged position by comparison with the NHS. This is justified given the difficult task they have to do, but on the other hand there are some aspects of NHS administration from whose adoption Rampton might benefit.

27.1.4   All the administrative and clerical staff at Rampton are civil servants whose only opportunity for direct experience of hospital administration is in one of the four special hospitals, the only hospitals directly managed by the DHSS. Comparable staff in the NHS are employees of Health Authorities and not civil servants. Despite the lack of opportunity they have had of training and experience in hospital management the Administrator and his staff at Rampton are capable and committed, and the service they provide is of a high order. On the other hand there is a well established profession of hospital and health administration with its own professional examinations, graduate and non-graduate training schemes and specialist courses and much greater use could be made of NHS experience in hospital administration to develop administration and financial systems at Rampton and in staff training. Another area where cross-fertilisation with the NHS would be useful would be in assessing work load, staff grading and staffing levels. Rampton's administrative and clerical staffing establishment is reviewed by DHSS staff inspectors at regular intervals, but it appears that the only comparisons which can be made are with other civil service offices. Comparisons with other psychiatric hospitals (apart from the other special hospitals) are not made because they are part of the NHS and do not therefore fall within the staff inspectors' remit. It should be made possible for there to be interchanges of staff between Rampton and the NHS and for NHS administrative staff to be seconded to Rampton. Professional meetings and training courses in the NHS should also be opened up to Rampton staff. Although it is not the concern of the Review Team it would of course be consistent to extend these opportunities to all special hospitals.

27.2 Observations on the various functions of the Administrator's department

27.2.1 The Administrator is graded as a principal and is assisted by three higher executive officers each of whom heads one of three staff sections; accommodation and supplies, medical records and finance. What follows is a brief review of the work currently undertaken, suggestions in connection with it and also proposals for the development and improvement of newer administrative functions.

27.2.2 Accommodation and supplies

Accommodation and maintenance as such are the responsibility of the Property Services Agency (PSA) of the Department of the Environment (see next Chapter), with whom this section of the Administrator's department liaises. The section is itself responsible for ordering supplies for the hospital—food, clothing, equipment, medical supplies etc—and appears to perform this function adequately and efficiently. The section also looks after the hospital housing estate. The estate is extensive and old fashioned and has in recent years been subject to various plans for modernisation or replacement. It appears that plans have been prepared, questioned, and fresh plans commissioned and this has led to delay and uncertainty. Many of the houses are unsatisfactory and a decision should be made soon for their phased improvement or replacement.

27.2.3 Medical records and information

Patients' records at Rampton are exceptionally well kept, thorough, well-documented and well compiled, and are an example to many hospitals. The medical records section also keeps account of the current validity of Mental Health Act orders to which all patients are subject, handles all documentation on patient movements, compiles hospital statistics, and services various officer committees. (This last function may need strengthening if, as we propose in paragraph 29.5.6, the Administrator is to service and be secretary of the proposed Review Board.) It is the section which compiles the data to inform Rampton management how its clinical work is changing and it is pleasing to see a developing interest in examining various aspects of hospital activity with the assistance of statistical information. It is surprising that Rampton and the other special hospitals are not required by DHSS to keep the same statistical information as NHS hospitals and this should be reviewed. There is a central Special Hospitals Research Unit run under DHSS auspices which should also have as part of its remit the presentation of information about the changing operational performance of the special hospitals. This is of particular importance in order to provide necessary background information for planning and policy decisions.

27.2.4 Finance and planning

We deal with wider aspects of finance and planning in Chapter 29. The finance department at Rampton is responsible for paying the large majority of staff and the general expenses of the hospital and once more the staff give the hospital an excellent service. We had one or two complaints that the physical remoteness of the department (in the old Superintendent's house on the estate) causes some inconvenience but it is clear that pay problems are in general dealt with promptly and sympathetically.

27.2.5 Personnel Management

In a number of respects personnel management and welfare functions seem under-developed at Rampton and given the hospital's history of difficulty some attention to this would seem essential. Both the Administrator and Chief Nursing Officer wish to develop a joint personnel department and every encouragement should be given to this development. There are two particular aspects of staff welfare which might be mentioned here. First of all, there are no clearly recognised arrangements at Rampton for the treatment of staff injured on duty: most treatment is provided either at the accident department at the nearest general hospital or by the person's own general practitioner. With as many doctors as there are at Rampton it should be possible for some form of emergency treatment service to be provided. Secondly, we think there should be a proper occupational health service at Rampton on the lines recommended in the Tunbridge Report* in 1968.

27.2.6 Press and public relations

If Rampton is to cast off its reputation as a 'secret hospital', it is important that it has a positive press and public relations policy. We deal with this specifically in paragraph 31.6.1. Public relations will be a major concern of the Review Board. At officer level however the Administrator has a particular responsibility in this area and advice and training should be made available.

27.2.7 Managing and co-ordinating the institutional services

We consider the institutional services at Rampton—catering, domestic services, portering, transport, laundry and supplies—in detail in the next Chapter. The heads of those services report directly to the Administrator. For an Administrator to be personally accountable for all these services he must be sure that the individual managers are clear what is expected of their

*Report of the Joint Committee on the Care of the Health of Hospital Staff. HMSO 1968.

departments and that they keep him informed of problems. In particular the standards of service achieved should be known to the Administrator by personal inspection and not simply by report. It is essential for him to be out and about, talking to staff and seeing for himself so that he is well informed about the current standards of their services and the general atmosphere of the hospital. It should be normal for the Administrator and his staff to be seen regularly in wards and departments. It is necessary for the Administrator to undertake a large part of this activity sampling personally, but one of his assistants should also have specifically delegated to him the task of overseeing the work of the institutional services.

CHAPTER 28

INSTITUTIONAL SERVICES

28.1 Introduction

28.1.1 Rampton's catering, domestic, maintenance and other housekeeping services are good and compare favourably with those in NHS psychiatric hospitals. Although not directly concerned with the care and treatment of patients they do make a valuable contribution to the quality of daily life at Rampton. The departments are well managed and we found evidence that the managers keep themselves informed of developments in their field and are prepared to adapt their services in response to changing needs of patients.

28.1.2 Selected posts in these departments are filled by patients and the realistic working conditions provide a valuable preparation and training for their eventual return to society. Recruitment is carried out by the occupations department who ensure that the job content is appropriate for rehabilitation purposes.

28.2 Catering

Patients' meals are prepared in the main kitchen situated within the hospital. Its equipment is modern and it provides a number of jobs for patients. The staff restaurant is outside the secure area and has its own kitchen. The service compares well with the standard of catering normally found in large institutions and finds favour with patients and staff. On one occasion Team members were present on a villa ward at lunch-time when the meal was not up to standard but the patients were most insistent that this was exceptional and that the food was one of the good features of life at Rampton. Praise was also given in private interviews with patients. The catering manager attends meetings of hospital caterers in the Trent NHS Region and keeps himself informed of developments. He and his staff visit wards at mealtimes and are steadily extending a choice of menu to all wards.

28.3 Domestic Services

The standard of cleanliness of the accommodation at Rampton is admirable. Much of the cleaning, particularly on the male block wards, is still done by patients supervised by nursing staff, as used to be the general rule in NHS psychiatric hospitals until recent years. Domestic staff clean the female wards, corridors and offices; the domestic manager employs and trains patients working in teams to clean other areas of the hospital using appropriate modern techniques and equipment. The manager inspects the domestic cleaning of the hospital regularly and we were pleased to note some changes and improvements introduced in the last year, notably the introduction of a complete steam-cleaning service for Victoria Ward (which has special problems—see paragraph 12.4).

28.4 Maintenance Services

Rampton enjoys an investment in maintenance services far exceeding that in the NHS and by any standards the service is good. The works staff are employed not by DHSS but by the PSA, which is responsible for maintaining all Government property. The local management and staff are based at Rampton and although they also look after a nearby prison and some Government offices, they have a very real loyalty to the hospital and the works officer is concerned to provide as good a service as possible. Like most works departments it is criticised by nursing and other staff for a lack of prompt response to requests for repairs or maintenance, but a check we did on completion of works requisitions conducted over a period of a month gave little support to such criticism. Rampton is exceptional in having a night maintenance engineer regularly on site as well as an 'on call' service at night and at weekend for other trades and this indicates the standards provided and expected at the hospital.

28.5 Transport

This service was until recently also provided by PSA but responsibility has now been transferred to the Administrator's department. A new and larger transport department has been set up complete with a fleet of new vehicles. We foresee the transport department taking an active role in organising and co-ordinating the transport for patients' visitors (see paragraph 31.3.4) as well as perhaps providing more opportunity for outings for patients and the increase in the number of drivers and vehicles will enable the department to undertake this additional work.

28.6 Clothing, linen and laundry

28.6.1   Patients may obtain clothing either by purchase in the hospital shop or on issue from the hospital. Many items for issue are made by patients in the hospital, men's clothing in the tailors' workshop and women's clothing in the sewing room. Many psychiatric hospitals operate their clothing stores in the style of an ordinary shop where patients have facilities to select and try on clothing; we think something similar might be of value at Rampton. However, if the methods of issuing clothing are somewhat traditional, certainly the range and variety available are first class and those responsible for this service demonstrate a commendable sensitivity and imagination. Clothing can be a powerful method of institutionalising patients. This certainly does not happen at Rampton, except to the extent that, as has been remarked elsewhere in this report, there is a tendency to insist on a greater formality in dress than in contempory society, for example, the wearing of ties.

28.6.2   The laundry provides a very good service to the hospital and useful work experience to the female patients who form the majority of staff. We recommend that all items of hospital issue clothing should be allocated to patients on a personal basis.

28.7 Porters and Car Park Attendants

We heard more genuine but small and apparently soluble complaints from this group of staff than from the others in the institutional services. Some of these have since been resolved. The morale of this group of staff would be improved however if they felt that somebody was listening to and trying to deal with their problems. A regular meeting with a designated member of the administrative staff would be valuable and this should be arranged by local management.

28.8 The Patients' Shop

28.8.1   The patients' shop is a much appreciated amenity, particularly for the longer-stay patients. It offers a varied range of goods; some two-thirds of the turnover is on tobacco and sweets but patients can also buy radios, clothes, toilet sundries, games, ornaments and many other things.

28.8.2   The shop-keeper and his staff provide a kind and helpful service in very poor conditions. The shop is an internal room with sky-lights and no windows situated off one of the main corridors; it is too small for the job it has to do. Working conditions are cramped, the shop is badly ventilated and heated, and there is no lavatory. We recommend that new and much larger accommodation be provided for the shop with improved facilities for the staff, and perhaps some self-service facilities for patients.

28.8.3   Apart from the specific question of accommodation, we think the hospital should institute a general review of its policy on the shop. Such a review would have to decide on the shop's purpose, whether it was intended simply to provide an amenity or whether it should contribute to rehabilitation by keeping patients in touch with one aspect of life in the outside world. Prices are far cheaper than those outside because mark-up is restricted, and although this provides value for money, patients tend to lose touch with current prices. At present the majority of patients have the opportunity of a monthly visit to the shop and at weekly intervals in between they may send written orders; this arrangement appears inflexible particularly for those being trained for departure. All transactions are by credit transfer since patients are not allowed to handle money. We think that there is a case for allowing patients before discharge or transfer to practice using money again, even if they are not permitted to take it on the wards and indeed we see no reason why pre-discharge patients as well as using the patients' shop should not make use of the post office and general store provided for staff in the hospital grounds.

CHAPTER 29

MANAGEMENT, FINANCE AND PLANNING

29.1 Introduction

In Chapter 6 we gave a brief account of our proposals for changes in the way Rampton is managed. We outlined our recommendations for a three-man Hospital Management Team at Rampton, led by a Medical Director, with responsibility for day-to-day management; a Heads of Department Committee with reponsibilities for the planning of policy and resource allocation; and a Review Board appointed for a period of three years to ensure that the proposals in our report are implemented and with wide supervisory powers over the running of the hospital. In this chapter we explain further why we think these changes in Rampton's management structure are necessary, give more detail about how we envisage the new structure would work in practice, and comment on the financial and planning procedures at Rampton, with suggestions as to how they might operate under the new structure.

29.2 The present management arrangements at Rampton (see figure A)

29.2.1   The management and control of Rampton is vested in the Secretary of State for Social Services. The Secretary of State exercises these responsibilities directly and not, as in the case of NHS hospitals, through the medium of statutorily established Health Authorities. In practice, this responsibility is exercised through the agency of DHSS, which the Secretary of State heads. Administrative aspects of the management of the special hospitals are the major concern of one branch ('MHC') of the DHSS Mental Health Division headed by an assistant secretary. Two principals and 22 more junior executive and clerical staff are exclusively employed on special hospital matters. There are doctors, nurses and social workers on the DHSS staff who are also concerned with special hospital management, though they all have other responsibilities as well. DHSS have set up a central management body for the special hospitals, called the Special Hospitals Office Committee (SHOC). Its membership is flexible, but always includes the assistant secretary in charge of MHC and the appropriate senior professionals. It is chaired by the under secretary in charge of the Mental Health Division. SHOC does not meet at set times, but as and when necessary. It makes formal visits to the special hospitals twice a year. The members are not formally appointed but hold office by virtue of their DHSS responsibilities. There is no statutory definition of SHOC's constitution or role nor any formal delegation of functions. It does not keep any formal record of its meetings, other than those with management and staff representatives at the hospitals held in the course of the twice-yearly visits.

29.2.2   At hospital level, the management at Rampton Hospital has suffered a number of vicissitudes over the past ten years, which need to be briefly described. Until 1972 the management responsibility had for many years been vested solely in the post of Medical Superintendent. However, following a HAS recommendation a Hospital Committee was established in 1972 to discuss hospital policy on multi-disciplinary basis. The Committee was chaired by the Medical Superintendent, who remained responsible for day-to-day

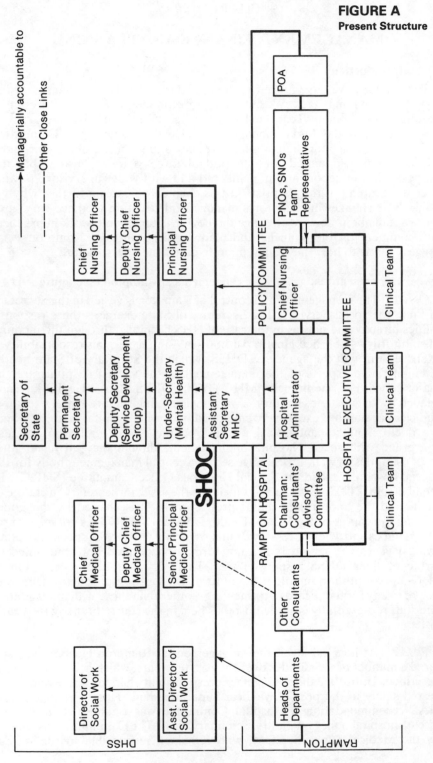

FIGURE A
Present Structure

→ Managerially accountable to
----- Other Close Links

SHOC

DHSS

RAMPTON

Secretary of State
Permanent Secretary
Deputy Secretary (Service Development Group)
Under-Secretary (Mental Health)
Assistant Secretary MHC

Chief Nursing Officer
Deputy Chief Nursing Officer
Principal Nursing Officer

Chief Medical Officer
Deputy Chief Medical Officer
Senior Principal Medical Officer

Director of Social Work
Asst. Director of Social Work

POLICY COMMITTEE

POA
PNOs, SNOs Team Representatives
Chief Nursing Officer

RAMPTON HOSPITAL
Hospital Administrator
Chairman: Consultants' Advisory Committee
Other Consultants
Heads of Departments

HOSPITAL EXECUTIVE COMMITTEE
Clinical Team
Clinical Team
Clinical Team
Clinical Team

116

management decisions; it compromised heads of all professional disciplines and two representatives of the nursing staff. A member of DHSS staff attended meetings as an observer.

29.2.3   Before this arrangement had time to have much effect a serious breakdown in management/staff relations occurred in the autumn of 1972 over an attempt to impose a new shift system on nurses, and Mr James Elliott was asked to carry out his enquiry (see paragraph 3.4). His report included a suggestion that the overall management of the hospital should be vested in a governing body of people drawn from outside the hospital and from DHSS. In the discussions which followed it became clear that the staff did not wish to be removed from direct management by DHSS; the Department also saw difficulties and the recommendation was not therefore acted on. Instead the post of Medical Superintendent was abolished and a part-time Medical Director was appointed in January 1974 for two years; he had no clinical responsibilities but acted in a general administrative capacity and chaired an extended committee—the Hospital Executive Team.

29.2.4   These arrangements encountered criticism in the hospital; the nursing staff felt under-represented whilst others felt that the Hospital Executive Team was too large a body to be able to carry out the day-to-day management of the hospital. The position of the Medical Director was also questioned. After considerable discussion in both DHSS and the hospital, the post of Medical Director was allowed to lapse in 1976, and the present management structure was introduced. It is based primarily on two main bodies, the Hospital Policy Committee and the Hospital Executive Committee.

29.2.5   The Hospital Policy Committee is formally responsible to DHSS for the formulation of policy at the hospital within the broad policy and guidance laid down by DHSS. It has 30 members, consisting of senior hospital staff from all disciplines, staff association representatives and two representatives from each clinical team (see 29.2.7 below). The Chairman is from DHSS (the assistant secretary in MHC).

29.2.6   The Hospital Executive Committee is formally responsible to the Policy Committee for the implementation of agreed policies and for day-to-day management. It consists of the Hospital Administrator, the Chairman of the Consultants Advisory Committee and the Chief Nursing Officer (all of whom are also members of the Policy Committee). Other Heads of Departments—the Principal Psychologist, the Principal Social Worker, the Chief Occupations Officer and the Senior Education Officer—are co-opted onto the Executive Committee as necessary and all Heads of Departments exercise day-to-day responsibility for the management of their own departments. Since 1978 there have been constant problems, which we described in detail in Chapter 16, about medical representation on the Executive Committee; the present arrangements were introduced only in November 1979 (after we had started work at the hospital).

29.2.7   The clinical services of the hospital are organised on a multi-disciplinary team basis. The hospital is divided into three areas (two male, one female). The multi-disciplinary team for each area consists of two or three consultants (one of whom takes the chair), a medical assistant, a senior nursing officer, three unit nursing officers, charge nurses/ward sisters and ward staff from up to 12 wards, two or more social workers, a psychologist, a teacher, a senior occupations officer and a deputy administrator. Each team meets from time to time to consider area policy. It also considers any matters concerning hospital policy as a whole referred for consideration by the Executive or the Policy Committee; to that extent teams have a role beyond clinical matters within their own area and are part of the consultative or policy-making mechanism of the hospital as a whole.

29.3 Our criticisms of the present management structure

29.3.1 The status of SHOC as the body managing the special hospitals on behalf of the Secretary of State, is ambiguous and unclear. Historically SHOC was designed to take over many of the functions of the old Board of Control, from which responsibility for the special hospitals was transferred to the Secretary of State in 1960. But unlike the Board of Control (or a NHS authority) SHOC is not a body corporate, it has no formal legal standing, and its members are all civil servants. It is in fact merely an informal DHSS office committee. But DHSS tend sometimes to present SHOC as if it were a clearly defined management tier or indeed, like its predecessor, the Board of Control, some sort of 'authority' in its own right. This conceals the reality of the situation, which is that there is no one 'tier' of management responsible for the special hospitals above the level of the hospitals themselves: instead there are various hierarchies of DHSS officials (see figure A) with the Secretary of State himself at the apex and managers at the individual hospitals at the base, with SHOC providing only one of many formal and informal co-ordinating mechanisms between these hierarchies.

29.3.2 DHSS officials in London are far too involved with day-to-day management of Rampton. Individual officers are sometimes moved away from MHC to other posts in DHSS before they have had time to acquire the necessary expertise. In any case, Rampton can hardly be managed effectively at a range of 150 miles. We think over-involvement by DHSS has largely arisen not because of empire building on the part of the Department but because of a lack of effective leadership at Rampton itself. But effective local leadership is hardly likely to emerge when at Rampton (uniquely amongst the special hospitals) the major policy making body, the Policy Committee, is chaired by an official from the DHSS in London.

29.3.3 There is no outside body which can scrutinise and comment on Rampton's activities on behalf of the wider public interest. Patients are at a disadvantage in that there is no readily accessible person or body of people to whom they can turn if they want a complaint or grievance investigated by an independent authority comparable by example to Boards of Visitors for prisoners or members of Health Authorities for patients in NHS hospitals.

29.3.4 The management structure at Rampton does not maintain a clear enough distinction between managerial accountability and responsibility on

118

the one hand and consultation and negotiation with staff on the other. This produces large and unwieldy 'talking shops' such as the Policy Committee (and its various subordinate committees) and the clinical teams which, although they have formal executive powers, in practice find it difficult to take decisions because they cannot arrive at anything approaching a consensus. The clear lines of accountability in the nursing hierarchy are disrupted by the fact that comparatively junior nurses are members of these bodies, as representatives of wards, teams or the POA, and appear to sit as peers and on occasion monitors of their senior officers.

29.3.5   There has been inadequate medical input into the management of the hospital. Mr Elliott identified this as a problem in 1973, and there has been little improvement since. We discussed the problems of medical organisation at Rampton in detail in Chapter 16.

29.3.6   There is no one person at Rampton to co-ordinate the management of the hospital as a whole and, if necessary, exercise a final arbitration before matters pass on to the next level.

29.3.7   Rampton lacks a spokesman to represent and, if necessary, defend the hospital in dealing with the outside world and in particular the media. The Secretary of State with the assistance of DHSS officials does his best to discharge this function but he must often be inhibited from speaking out by legal, constitutional or political considerations.

29.4   Our recommendations for a new management structure:

A. Internal management (For this and section 29.5 below, see figure B).

29.4.1   We think that local responsibility for the running of Rampton should in future be vested primarily in a Hospital Management Team (HMT) consisting of the Medical Director (see the next paragraph), the Chief Nursing Officer and the Administrator. As we explained in Chapter 6, its function would be to take day-to-day decisions affecting the hospital as a whole and to maintain a general oversight of implementation of agreed hospital policy.

29.4.2   We recommend in Chapter 16 that a Medical Director should be appointed at Rampton. Our objective is that the Medical Director in addition to his purely medical functions, should provide the overall co-ordination and leadership which Rampton so much needs. To reflect this role, we think he should be appointed ex-officio Chairman of the HMT for the first three years of his appointment. After that we think it would be right to adopt the normal NHS procedure and provide for the chairman to be elected by the HMT. As Chairman of the HMT, we would expect the Medical Director to take the lead in developing clinical and research policies at Rampton and ensuring that the functions of all departments of the hospital were properly co-ordinated. He would also be responsible for ensuring that standards of care were properly monitored.

29.4.3   We think there should be a Heads of Department Committee (HDC) consisting of the members of the HMT, the heads of the education, occupation, social work and psychology departments and the chairman of the

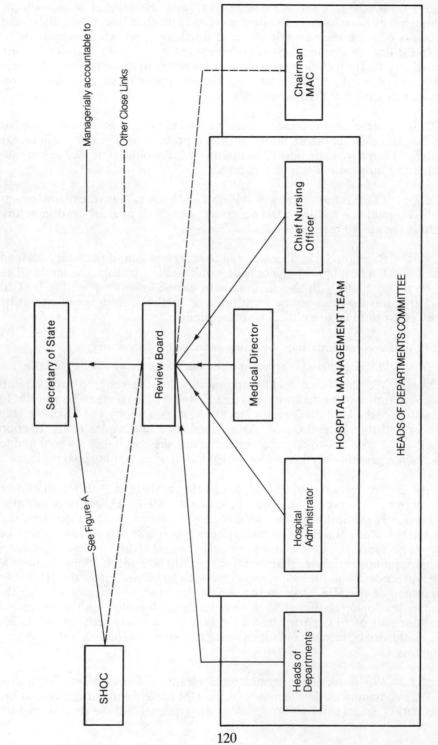

FIGURE B
Proposed Structure

Managerially accountable to
Other Close Links

Chairman MAC

Chief Nursing Officer

Secretary of State

Review Board

Medical Director

HOSPITAL MANAGEMENT TEAM

HEADS OF DEPARTMENTS COMMITTEE

See Figure A

Hospital Administrator

Heads of Departments

SHOC

120

Medical Advisory Committee (see paragraph 16.7.9). The PNO (Education) would attend as required. The HDC would have responsibility for
— the compilation of the annual operational plan;
— providing policy and planning directions for the hospital; and
— proposals for the allocation of resources amongst the various services at the hospital (see 29.6 and 29.7 below).
Throughout it would act subject to the directions and approval of the Review Board (see 29.5). It would provide a regular forum for the exchange of information and consultation with the HMT. The present Policy Committee would be abolished. It is large, unwieldy and ineffectual.

29.4.4   We think that the three clinical teams should continue to function, though attendance at meetings, particularly of nurses, could be reduced to more manageable proportions. Their main business should be to co-ordinate services for the care of the patients, and their involvement in the general management of the hospital should largely be limited to contributing proposals to the annual operational plan and commenting on it. Clinical teams should not be seen as a negotiating forum between management and staff, as they appear to be at present. Consultants should continue to chair the clinical teams and the administration should provide secretarial support. Teams should report to the HMT.

29.4.5   We recommend that in addition, for the reasons we discussed in Chapter 22, there should be a resocialisation team, also reporting to the HMT and comprising the heads of the education, psychology, occupations and social work departments, the SNO (Activities) and a doctor nominated by the Medical Advisory Committee. Its function would be to plan and co-ordinate the services offered by resocialisation departments to the clinical teams, to contribute to the annual operational plan and to comment upon it. The team should elect its own chairman and the administration should provide secretarial support.

29.4.6   We explained in Chapter 6 that in our view the POA or other staff associations should not be represented within the management structure, as this seems to us to confuse management with consultation (see also paragraph 29.3.4 above), but that instead there should be a joint committee of management and staff, which should meet at regular intervals with both sides contributing to the agenda. On the management side, the HMT would represent the management at the majority of meetings. The Review Board (see 29.5) would meet with the staff side at regular but less frequent intervals to discuss major matters or those where agreement could not be reached with the HMT. We think that arrangements of this sort could be devised without difficulty on the basis of the existing formal Whitley Council system and the current arrangements for informal regular discussions between the Hospital Executive and the POA executive.

29.4.7   We have proposed above the abolition of the Policy Committee and a reduction in the number of people attending clinical team meetings. We think both these proposals will clarify the responsibility of the hospital managers to manage and separate it from their responsibility to inform and consult their own staff. But the very fact that under our proposals fewer people will be directly and personally involved in the formulation of hospital and clinical team policies at the highest level makes it all the more important that top managers should ensure that their channels of communication (in both directions) with their own staff are working properly. In addition to good machinery for staff consultation there needs to be an effective system of communication within the hospital if things are to be understood and implemented. We recommend that the hospital should seek the help of a body like the Industrial Society, experienced in instituting effective communication systems.

29.5   Our recommendations for a new management structure

B.   A Review Board

29.5.1   We described in Chapter 6 why we thought Rampton needed a Review Board, what its membership should be and what in general terms its functions should be to ensure that the recommendations in our report are implemented and to provide a degree of public surveillance over the operations of the hospital. In this chapter we discuss these functions in a little more detail. We have not however attempted to provide a complete blueprint for how we think the Board should operate, or to describe in detail exactly how we think it should manage its relations with DHSS on the one hand and the management at Rampton on the other. Much of the detail must be left for future discussions between the DHSS, the hospital and the members of the Board.

29.5.2   We suggest that the Board should have formally delegated to it for a period of three years all the powers over and responsibilities towards Rampton which are at present exercised by the Secretary of State, with the exception of certain specified powers and responsibilities which would be reserved to the Secretary of State (see paragraph 29.5.3). The Secretary of State would retain reserve powers of direction over the Board, but the assumption would be that these would need to be used only in exceptional circumstances. The Board would however be expected to operate within any general policy guidelines laid down by DHSS for the special hospitals as a whole. The Board would be required to have regard in its work to the recommendations of the Review Team contained in this report and so far as possible to ensure that they were implemented. It would also be required to submit periodic reports on its work to the Secretary of State.

29.5.3   We think the Secretary of State would need to reserve specific powers in the following areas:

a.   *Staff.*   All staff at Rampton would remain civil servants and terms and conditions of service would continue to be negotiated centrally for all special hospital staff. We would envisage however that the Review Board would themselves make the most senior appointments (at a minimum the Medical Director, heads of departments and consultants), subject in each case to the approval of the Secretary of State.

b.   *Admissions, discharges and transfers.* We think that DHSS should retain control of admissions and that DHSS and the Home Office involvement in discharge and transfer (see Chapter 15) should remain as at present. (We said in paragraph 9.1.4 that we thought that Rampton

122

consultants should however be involved more often in the selection process.)

c.   *Financial and manpower allocations*. Rampton's overall manpower limits and revenue allocation would continue to be determined by DHSS and its capital allocation by PSA in consultation with DHSS (see section 29.6 below). The Board would of course put forward its views and proposals on these matters for approval by the DHSS.

29.5.4   We are advised that a Review Board for Rampton with the powers outlined in the preceding paragraphs could be constituted as a 'special health authority' by an Order under section 11 of the NHS Act 1977.

29.5.5   We discuss in the next chapter the role of the Review Board in the handling of complaints. There are other less formal ways in which Board members could provide the outside scrutiny over the working of the hospital which we think is an essential part of the Board's function. We would expect Board members to spend as much time as possible round and about the hospital, with the same sort of unrestricted access as we have had talking to the staff and patients, asking questions, and reporting back to the full Board as necessary. Each member might take on a special responsibility for some defined aspect of the hospital's work.

29.5.6   We visualise that the Board would meet monthly. It should be serviced by the hospital Administrator and his staff, the Administrator acting as its secretary. We think that the Administrator's staff would need to be augmented for this new role, probably by the appointment of a committee clerk. The other members of the HMT would normally attend meetings of the Board; other heads of departments would attend as required. The Chairman should have direct access to the Secretary of State.

29.5.7   We suggested in Chapter 6 that it would be desirable for there to be some link between the Board and the Review Team. This might be achieved by making one member of the Team a member of the Board—perhaps for a limited period; but there are other ways in which the knowledge and experience of the Team could be made available to the Board. In much the same way we think that arrangements should be made through which the knowledge and experience of DHSS officials could be made available to the Board, whether by invitation to attend Board meetings or otherwise.

29.6   Finance

29.6.1   The arrangements under which Rampton is financed are complicated. Rampton receives a share of the total resource allocation which DHSS negotiates with the Treasury and other central departments for the special hospitals as a whole and which is approved by the Government collectively. Salaries (£5.8 million at Rampton in 1979/80) and other revenue expenditure (£1.7 million in 1979/80) are the responsibility of DHSS. Expenditure on salaries is controlled largely by manpower limits agreed between DHSS and the Civil Service Department. Once DHSS have agreed the annual revenue budget and manpower limit for each hospital, they do not in general interfere with how each hospital uses its allocation. If however for any reason (for example, recruitment difficulties) one hospital is unable to take up its full allocation of money or manpower approvals DHSS are able to switch the unused portion to another hospital, and it appears that in the past Rampton has been a net beneficiary under this arrangement. Money for capital projects is operationally and for accounting purposes the responsibility of the Department of the Environment.

29.6.2   In general, it is clear that shortage of funds is not one of Rampton's problems. We are told that the special hospitals' position has been specially protected under the present Government's public expenditure policy. We have also been told however that a restriction of PSA's funds has caused some delay in minor building projects (ie up to £100,000) at the special hospitals, which have had to 'take their place in the queue' with other Departments' projects. We think the particular needs of the special hospitals should be recognised in the PSA's minor capital programme.

29.6.3   We do not envisage that the new management structure proposed earlier in this chapter should involve any substantial change in the financial arrangements at Rampton, except that the Review Board would clearly have to be involved in negotiating Rampton's share of the total special hospital budget with DHSS and in approving Rampton's own budget within the resources eventually allocated. The Administrator would continue to be the accounting officer for the hospital.

29.6.4   The system of internal budgetary control at Rampton is elementary and should be extended and improved as an early priority. There is little evidence of financial planning and many decisions with financial consequences are taken on an *ad hoc* basis with no attempt to distinguish between competing priorities. Advice from those responsible for operating similar procedures in the NHS might well be sought.

29.6.5   At present Rampton has a Finance Committee with members at below head of department level. We think this is unsatisfactory: in our view discussion by officers of resource allocation can in practice only take place at head of department level. Under the new management structure we think the HMT should be responsible for financial control, and the HDC for the allocation of resources and the preparation of the budget (subject to the approval of the Review Board).

29.7   Planning

Like the budgetary procedures, systematic strategic planning for Rampton (and indeed, so far as we can see, for the special hospitals as a whole) is at a very rudimentary stage. We have however been encouraged to note some recent progress in this area. At the request of DHSS, each department of the hospital has produced an individual policy and strategy statement, which we have had the opportunity of seeing. These statements contain many constructive and forward-looking ideas and anticipate many of our own suggestions. We think the next stage should be the development and agreement of a policy and strategy statement for the hospital as a whole. This could then be translated into an operational plan linked with the annual budget, and updated annually.

124

Again we hope this is something to which the Review Board and the HDC will give their early attention. The DHSS is currently revising and simplifying the planning systems for the NHS and as in the case of financial procedures (see paragraph 29.6.4) there would seem to be some advantage in obtaining advice from the NHS.

CHAPTER 30

COMPLAINTS

30.1 Our remit

Our terms of reference directed us to examine the procedures for complaints and the formulation of a system for making and dealing with complaints in line with the best current practice elsewhere. We were not asked to investigate particular complaints and indeed were specifically precluded from collecting or considering any allegations of deliberate ill treatment of patients as these matters were being examined by the police for the Director of Public Prosecutions. As we have mentioned in paragraph 1.3, we did not come across any evidence of ill treatment of patients; we received one letter containing fresh allegations of ill-treatment, from an ex-patient and this we passed to the police.

30.2 The position prior to May 1979

Prior to May 1979 the normal procedure for dealing with complaints received at the hospital was that the Administrator would arrange for an investigation to be carried out by senior staff in the discipline concerned. Thus any complaint about nursing staff would be investigated by other more senior nurses. A report would then be made to the Administrator, who was responsible for ensuring that the investigation had been properly and adequately conducted. The Administrator would then arrange for a reply to be sent to the complainant or, if the original complaint has been received by DHSS and passed to the hospital for investigation, would make a report to DHSS. A summary of complaints was kept in the Administrator's office and was inspected periodically by a senior officer from DHSS.

30.2.2 We carried out an analysis of complaints dealt with under these arrangements during a five year period, January 1974 to December 1978. There were a total of 178 complaints: 71 in 1974; 46 in 1975; 30 in 1976; 18 in 1977; and 13 in 1978. We were unable to discover any conclusive explanation for the steady fall in the number of complaints. The introduction of villa visiting for patients' friends and families and the encouragement of charge nurses/ward sisters on block wards to meet patients' families at visiting time, thereby possibly resolving problems and complaints by personal contact, may have been a contributory factor.

30.2.3 We classified complaints according to the subject raised: of the 178, 52 were allegations of cruelty to patients by staff; 10 were complaints of cruelty to patients by other patients; 28 were complaints about visiting arrangements (distance, cost, lack of refreshment facilities, delays on arrival and cancellation at short notice); and 88 were miscellaneous complaints such as lack of information about decisions to transfer or change of medication, loss of property and failure to receive mail. Complaints appear to be fairly evenly distributed among patient groups: 54 complaints concerned mental illness patients; 52 concerned psychopathic patients; 55 concerned mentally handicapped patients and 17 concerned severely mentally handicapped patients. Some patients and some families lodged a large number of complaints: the families of three patients made six complaints each and seven patients account for 32 complaints.

30.2.4   In carrying out our analysis, we examined a number of complaint files. Matters appeared to have been investigated in detail, and thorough, well-drafted replies were sent to complainants. On the other hand, we were surprised to discover that of the 178 complaints received during the period, not one had been substantiated. In this connection, we noted the information about disciplinary proceedings at special hospitals given by Sir George Young, Parliamentary Under-Secretary of State at the DHSS, in reply to a Parliamentary Question on 16 January 1980. This was to the effect that during the three years 1976–1978 formal disciplinary proceedings against staff at Broadmoor were taken on 15 occasions, at Moss Side on nine occasions, at Park Lane on four occasions, but not at all at Rampton. There is clearly room for argument about how these figures should be interpreted, but in our view they must cast doubt on the effectiveness of the procedure for investigating complaints which was in operation at Rampton during the period in question.

30.3   The position between May 1979 and July 1980

During the period when police were investigating allegations of ill-treatment of patients arising from the television programme 'The Secret Hospital', it was decided by DHSS that all complaints which alleged ill-treatment of patients, of however trivial a nature, should not be investigated by the hospital but referred direct to the police. Other complaints were dealt with *ad hoc* by the Administrator.

30.4   Proposals for a revised procedure

30.4.1   Since 1978 the DHSS has been negotiating centrally with the staff of the special hospitals about a new procedure for dealing with complaints alleging physical ill-treatment of patients and, we assume, other serious complaints which would apply to all four hospitals. (It is accepted that this would be an interim procedure which might need amending when decisions have been taken on the adoption of a standard complaints procedure in the NHS, on which discussions are still proceeding following the report of the Davies Committee.) A revised procedure, which seemed to us to be in general satisfactory, was in fact agreed by the staff at all the special hospitals except Rampton and came into operation in January 1979, but we understand that the POA centrally have subsequently raised objections to it and advised their members in all the special hospitals not to operate it. Although we are told that POA branches have not always followed this advice, to all intents and purposes there is at present no agreed procedure for dealing with serious complaints at any of the four special hospitals, including Rampton.

30.4.2   The procedure adopted in the other special hospitals in 1979 provided that investigation into complaints alleging physical ill-treatment of patients should be carried out by a team of two or three people appointed by the Hospital Management Team (HMT) or equivalent body. The investigation team would comprise a senior member of the discipline to which the complaint related, and one or two senior members of other disciplines. The investigation team would report to the HMT who would decide on further action. If the HMT were satisfied that there was a prima facie case that ill-treatment of a more than minor nature had occurred, they would consider whether the matter should be reported to the police.

30.4.3   We understand that the principal POA objections to this procedure, which led to them advising their members not to operate it, are twofold. First of all, they think that complaints against nurses should be investigated solely by nurses, or at any rate that nurses should have a clear majority on any investigating panel. We cannot agree with this view. We think that an investigation conducted on the basis the POA suggest would not provide for the degree of impartiality which patients and public have the right to expect. It is important that justice is done and seen to be done. Best practice in the NHS is for serious complaints against nurses to be investigated by a doctor, an administrator and a nurse. In some instances, Health Authority members are also involved.

30.4.4   Secondly, we understand the POA are concerned that under the procedure the fact that a complaint has been internally investigated does not prevent the subsequent involvement of the police. They point to the fact that following 'The Secret Hospital' television programme, complaints which had already been investigated and rejected under an internal procedure were re-investigated by the police. This, they claim, puts their members in 'double jeopardy'. Morever, they fear that if the hospital management are able to refer complaints to the police when they have been partially investigated under the internal procedure and prima facie evidence of criminal offence has been found, the police may be able to make use of any statements which have been obtained in the course of the internal investigation without a formal caution having been administered. The POA therefore take the view that *all* complaints alleging ill-treatment of patients should be referred direct to the police, or at any rate that the person complained of should be given an option for the complaint to be referred to the police if he wishes.

30.4.5   We have some sympathy with the POA on this point, although we think that they underestimate the consequences of fairly regular and sometimes lengthy investigations by the police at the hospital if every complaint had to be dealt with by the police. We certainly think it is undesirable in normal circumstances that a complaint which has been fully investigated internally and found to have no substance should be subsequently referred to the police and in effect re-opened. (The present situation at Rampton, arising out of the allegations in 'The Secret Hospital', is abnormal and must we think be accepted as such.) We would also think it wrong that the police should be able to make use of any statements made in the course of an internal investigation without a caution having been administered (if in fact this could ever happen). But we think that management must have the right to decide whether a complaint should be referred initially to the police or considered under the internal procedure. There will always be cases where it appears that a criminal offence may technically have been committed but the police may decide for a variety of reasons that it does not warrant criminal proceedings. Such cases might nevertheless raise important issues of discipline or professional conduct on the part of staff and therefore warrant internal investigation by the hospital. Nor do we think that the decision to refer the complaint initially to the police or to consider it internally should be irreversible. After a case has been referred to them the police might decide that it should not be proceeded with but in such cases again an internal investigation might nonetheless be appropriate. Moreover, if the case is initially referred for internal investigation and it subsequently appears prima facie that ill-treatment may have occurred, we think it is right (subject to what we said earlier in this paragraph about statements obtained without a caution) that the case should be referred to the police.

30.4.6   We think therefore that the procedure for dealing with complaints at Rampton should reflect the following principles:

a. An internal hospital investigation is appropriate if the allegations, if proved true, would amount to a trivial or technical breach of the law, although they might conceivably raise serious questions of professional conduct or discipline. A police investigation is appropriate if there are serious allegations or if a complex and lengthy investigation is clearly needed into a complaint of a fairly serious character. It should be accepted that what started off in one way may finish in another. The police may remit a matter to management or management to the police, after initial investigation.

b. The most important aspect of any internal investigation is that it is seen to be impartial. In the Rampton context this seems to us to mean that any internal investigation must be multi-disciplinary.

c. We also think it should be made clear that the procedure is not concerned only with complaints which allege physical ill-treatment of patients but with all complaints other than the most trivial.

In general, the aim should be to ensure that those who wish to complain about Rampton can be assured that their complaint is dealt with no less sympathetically, impartially and efficiently than in the best NHS hospitals.

30.5   The role of the Review Board in the complaints procedure

We referred briefly in the previous chapter to the role of the proposed Review Board in the complaints procedure. In general we see the Review Board as taking over most of the DHSS's current functions with regard to complaints. If (and we hope this will not be the case) a satisfactory national agreement on complaints procedure has not been reached by the time the Review Body is set up we would expect them to take-over negotiations with the Rampton staff on a procedure for Rampton alone. We would expect the Review Board to monitor carefully all complaints received and satisfy themselves that agreed procedures were being properly applied. They would not be directly involved with the investigation of individual complaints except perhaps that a member of the Board might in serious cases warranting internal investigation sit as a member of the investigating panel. If however a complainant was dissatisfied with the outcome of an investigation by management at the hospital, it would be open to him to ask the Board to review the way the case had been handled. The Board would then have to decide what action, if any, should be taken.

CHAPTER 31

PATIENTS, THEIR RELATIVES AND THE OUTSIDE WORLD

31.1 Introduction

31.1.1 In this final chapter of our report, we make some suggestions which relate to different areas of Rampton's work but which have closely related objectives. They are all aimed at ensuring that in one way or another information about Rampton is more widely available and that its operations are opened up, to the maximum possible extent consistent with security, to the scrutiny of the outside world. The Yorkshire TV film which led to our being set up was called 'The Secret Hospital', an unfair title in some ways but nevertheless not in our view wholly inappropriate. Making sure that more people are properly informed about Rampton and understand its problems and achievements is vital to its future health as an institution as well as very much in the interests of patients, relatives and staff.

31.1.2 In this chapter we consider first of all how information is given to patients about the way Rampton works and the sort of treatment they can expect to receive. We then discuss the provision of information to relatives and the arrangements which are made for them to visit the hospital, to see the patients and discuss their treatment. We consider the restrictions which are placed on communications by letter and telephone between patients and their friends and relatives. Next we discuss the role of other visitors to Rampton, official and voluntary, and the chaplaincy arrangements; and finally we consider the hospital's relations with the media and the implications of the Official Secrets Act. But one of our most important specific suggestions in this field is one which has implications extending beyond Rampton and which we are therefore unable to develop in detail. This is the recommendation we made in paragraph 4.7, that consideration should be given to the establishment of a body to inspect and monitor all institutions where patients are subject to detention under the Mental Health Act.

31.2 Information given to patients

31.2.1 Soon after admission to Rampton, patients are officially 'briefed' about Rampton by the charge nurse on the admission ward. Patients are also given a formal notice explaining their legal status under the Mental Health Act and their rights to appeal to the MHRT and to apply for discharge to the hospital managers. A social worker visits all patients as soon as possible after admission to explain these rights, to ensure that any necessary immediate action is taken, eg on appeals, and to discuss family contacts which the social worker will be expecting to have. But we think that in addition there is a need for a simple and informally written booklet which could be issued to all patients soon after admission, explaining the practical aspects of life at Rampton and how the 'system' works. (Oral explanations by staff would still be necessary, particularly of course in the case of illiterate patients.) We have seen a copy of such a booklet produced at Rampton in 1972 which we thought was generally along the right lines; it appears however that for some reason it has not been issued to patients for some years and is now out of print. We recommend that it should be urgently revised and reprinted, and that steps should be taken to ensure that it is given to all new patients.

31.3 Facilities for patients' relatives

31.3.1 We think that Rampton should give a rather higher priority than it has in the past to meeting the needs of patients' relatives. Relatives should be given as much opportunity as possible of keeping in close touch with patients. They should be able to obtain full information about their progress and, if they wish, to discuss treatment and any other matters with the appropriate staff at the hospital. Regular contact with relatives can often help patients' progress; it can also help staff, by enabling misunderstandings or potential complaints to be resolved informally at an early stage.

31.3.2 When a patient is first admitted, his nearest relative is sent a booklet 'Information for the Guidance of Relatives and Friends'. It gives information about visiting arrangements and some other matters (including advice on how to make a complaint). We think this booklet is good in itself, although more information could usefully be included, particularly about the sort of life the patient will be leading in Rampton with some details of the educational, occupational and recreational facilities available. To supplement this written information, we suggest that there could be organised guided tours of the hospital from time to time, with introductory talks from senior staff and opportunities for questions, to which the relatives of recently admitted patients should be specifically invited. Well thought-out arrangements of this kind would be of great value to relatives.

31.3.3 Normal visiting times are every Saturday and Sunday, and the first and third Monday in each month, although relatives can visit at other times by prior arrangement. At present all patients see their visitors in the main recreational hall in the inner security area. Until June 1979, most male and some female patients were allowed to see their visitors on the villas. This had what seems to us the great advantage of allowing relatives to see and meet the nurses who were actually looking after the patients and to discuss with them any worries or problems. However in June 1979 when police enquiries were about to start following 'The Secret Hospital' television programme, nursing staff, for reasons which are not wholly clear to us, decided that they would no longer permit villa visiting. At the time of writing, it appears that the POA would be prepared to let villa visiting be resumed if an SNO were always on duty at the weekend visiting times to deal with any complaints which relatives might make about patients' treatment, but that the hospital management do not accept that this is necessary. We were surprised that this impasse has been allowed to continue so long. We urge the early reintroduction of villa visiting and its extention to all the female as well as all the male villas.

31.3.4 Rampton's geographical remoteness and its national catchment area create travelling difficulties for visitors. Retford railway station is six miles from Rampton, and there is only an infrequent bus service between the station and the hospital. On Monday visiting days and two Sundays out of four a coach hired by the hospital takes visitors without charge to and from

132

the station; we have had some complaints about the reliability of this service. On Saturdays visitors have to use the local bus service; this involves a long walk from the station to the bus stop and from the Rampton bus stop to the hospital. There is no local bus service on Sunday, so on those Sundays when the hospital does not provide a coach, visitors have to travel to the hospital by taxi. The hospital League of Friends organise long distance coaches to Rampton from various parts of the country during the summer months (at a nominal charge or none at all), with some financial help from DHSS. A 'self-help' coach is also organised from the south west of England in co-operation with local volunteers and social workers. Now that Rampton has its own transport department (see paragraph 28.5) and there is provision for an increase in vehicles and drivers we think the transport manager should, as part of his duties, co-ordinate all patients' and visitors' transport. He should look to needs where there are a number of visitors from a particular area and arrange transport by hiring it, by getting help from voluntary bodies or relatives' associations, or by using the hospital's own transport where appropriate.

31.3.5 Visitors who are receiving supplementary benefit can get the full cost of their travel to and from Rampton reimbursed; other visitors get half the cost repaid. But only the cost of travel by public transport can be reimbursed; visitors who travel by private car can claim nothing. We do not believe this restriction can be defended given the difficulties and cost of getting to Rampton by public transport, and we strongly recommend that the travel concessions are extended to travel by private car.

31.3.6 Facilities at the hospital itself are inadequate for visitors who may have had to travel a long way. There is little or no suitable overnight accommodation nearby and visitors cannot even obtain meals at the hospital. Visitors accompanied by children might welcome the provision of a creche. Following our discussions at the hospital the Administrator is circulating all relatives with a questionnaire to try to assess potential demand for such facilities, so that action can be taken to provide them where necessary. We hope this project will bear fruit.

31.3.7 Because of the difficulties over transport and accommodation, we do not think it would be practicable at this time to extend regular visiting hours beyond what they are at present (for example, to have regular visiting every afternoon), as has been suggested to us. As indicated above, relatives can visit 'out of hours' by prior arrangement. With better facilities, some extension of regular visiting times may be possible later.

31.4 Postal and telephone arrangements

31.4.1. One important way in which patients maintain their contacts with the world outside is by sending and receiving mail. All incoming and outgoing post is examined by a small staff of censors. There are exceptions to this interception as stipulated by section 36 of the Mental Health Act 1959; for example, patients may write direct to the Secretary of State or to any Member of Parliament. The reasons for censoring mail include the need to maintain security, to be aware of news which may seriously upset a patient, to avoid nuisance to patients or their correspondents, and to provide an independent check on the contents of parcels. The staff who undertake this work do so with understanding and sympathy. There are some occasions when post is returned to the sender or other action taken, for example when a patient writes to a mail order firm requesting tools or knives, but these are very rare. Whilst there is a need for this function, its application to all mail is increasingly recognised as unnecessary. Some patients could be excluded from its scope, for example some of the elderly, those about to leave Rampton, and patients who have demonstrated sufficiently responsible behaviour. In the past the possibility of introducing a measure of flexibility along the lines outlined above was discussed but rejected by staff. We believe that the proposed measures were sensible and did not undermine security, and we recommend that they should be introduced.

31.4.2   The telephone provides another useful link between patients and their families. Patients are not normally allowed to telephone but last year this rule was relaxed at Christmas. We welcome this and recommend that in appropriate cases patients should be allowed to use the telephone more freely.

31.5   Other visitors to Rampton

31.5.1   A number of voluntary bodies are closely connected with Rampton, providing an extremely useful service and also helping to bring the hospital more contact with the outside world. Firstly there is the League of Friends of Rampton. Their principal function is raising money to provide transport for relatives visiting from long distances (see paragraph 31.3.4 above). They have also provided the hospital with cine, photographic and disco equipment and a small sum of money for emergency use for patient needs by social workers. They are currently concerned with providing some special facilities for the disabled, particularly horse riding in co-operation with the National Society for Mentally Handicapped Children and a local horse owner. The Friends hope to start outings on a barge for some patients and are prepared to assist in equipping a social club for pre-discharge patients. They played a part in the setting up of most successful exhibitions of occupations department work in Retford and more recently in Lincoln Cathedral. Encouraging local enthusiasm and raising money for a hospital with a national catchment area is difficult; we commend the League for the excellent work they do and hope that it will be strongly encouraged and supported.

31.5.2   Representatives of the Townswomen's Guild visit female patients once a month and provide them with friendly contact. The hospital social work department in co-operation with the local authority social services department has been running a course for four to five prospective volunteers and it is hoped that they will become regular visitors to Rampton, particularly to those patients who have no family or friends. In some cases they will be able to provide a link with a patient's own family. Visits by professional and other groups for information and educational purposes are numerous. There were 295 during 1979. Some patients may well resent being 'stared at' but we feel that these visits are valuable to Rampton in that they enable more people to learn about the way the hospital works. There are also occasional visits by groups who come into the hospital for sports activities such as football, hockey, darts, badminton, basketball, rounders and table tennis against teams composed of patients. All these groups should be encouraged and where possible new ones invited; they make a very valuable contribution to the quality of life in an institution, especially in the case of long-stay patients.

31.5.3   The Worksop and Retford Community Health Council have no statutory responsibilities towards Rampton, as it is outside the NHS. Following the showing of 'The Secret Hospital' they were invited to visit the hospital whenever they chose and without notice. We understand that three or four such visits have already been made.

31.5.4   The Disablement Resettlement Officer (DRO) from the Manpower Commission visits regularly not only to lecture staff on the work of the Commission, but also to take part in pre-discharge discussion groups with patients and to see individually all patients before discharge to discuss employment, further training and liaison with the DRO in the area where the patients will be going.

31.5.5   Patients also of course receive visits from professional visitors such as solicitors and probation officers.

31.5.6   We believe that members of the Review Board will individually and collectively have an important role to play in developing all these contacts with the outside world and in guiding all aspects of the external relationships of the hospital.

31.6   Chaplaincy arrangements

Rampton's chaplaincy arrangements are similar to those of NHS hospitals. There is a full time Anglican chaplain on the staff and Roman Catholic, Free Church and other denominations are represented by visiting chaplains. Their work, both in the newly built chapel and on ward visits, is appreciated by both patients and staff.

31.7   Relations with the news media and the Official Secrets Act

31.7.1   In the past, Rampton has tended to be suspicious of the news media. Since we began our work, there have been some signs of a change of attitude which we welcome. We think Rampton has everthing to gain from enlisting the help of the media in projecting the positive aspects of its work to the general public and spreading a wider understanding of the problems it has to face. Conversely, of course, when things go seriously wrong, it must be accepted that there is a legitimate interest in bringing the facts to the attention of the public. In either case, an obstructive and suspicious attitude almost invariably results in a bad press. We think that, subject to security considerations and the need to protect individual patients' privacy, Rampton should offer the media every possible facility. Here again, we think that the Review Board should take the lead in encouraging openness, not only with the press but the public as well, for example, by promoting Open Days and the like. We think the media themselves should in return be prepared to report Rampton in a straightforward and balanced way.

31.7.2   Rampton's 'secretiveness' has often been linked with the provisions

135

of Section 2 of the Official Secrets Act which prohibits the disclosure of all official information to unauthorised persons and to which Rampton staff, as persons who hold 'office under Her Majesty' are automatically subject. In the context of the more open management style we have recommended, we think that less emphasis can and should be placed on the provisions of the Official Secrets Act which are in practice unlikely to have to be invoked save in exceptional cases such as those involving the disclosure of the security arrangements at the hospital.

31.7.3   Rampton staff have at present to seek prior permission of DHSS before delivering any lecture or publishing any article relating to their official duties. This is unnecessarily restrictive and encourages a closed approach by staff. Any necessary restrictions (for example on confidentiality of personal information about patients or security measures) should be clearly defined and staff should have to do no more than seek the approval of their head of department. Heads of departments and consultants should be left to use their own discretion about consulting the DHSS (or under the management arrangements we are proposing, The Review Board) if controversial issues may arise. Moreover we think that staff should be positively encouraged to give factual talks to local and professional organisations about the hospital and to write about their professional work in journals.

LIST OF RECOMMENDATIONS AND SUGGESTIONS

The wider context of our review and the future of Rampton

1.   DHSS should consider whether a wider review of the future role of special hospitals is called for. (Paragraph 4.2)

2.   We do not believe that Rampton should be closed. (Paragraph 4.6)

3.   DHSS should give consideration to the case for an appointed body to inspect and monitor all institutions where patients are subject to detention under the Mental Health Act. (Paragraph 4.7)

4.   The eventual aim should be to reduce the size of Rampton to 500 or 600 beds. (Paragraph 5.11)

The 'Rampton system'

5.   The future role of the Rampton Ethics Committee in monitoring some of the potential dangers of the 'system' should be reviewed. (Paragraph 7.2.4)

6.   Attempts to achieve a better streaming or 'peer-grouping' arrangement on more wards should be pursued more energetically. (Paragraph 7.3.1)

7.   Each patient should have a properly designed individual treatment programme. (Paragraph 7.3.2). Many patients would benefit from behaviour modification, self-care and social skills programmes including ward-based programmes run by nursing staff. Urgent steps should be taken to increase the clinical psychology involvement in treatment programmes. (Paragraph 7.3.3—see also recommendation 136 below)

8.   There should be further careful extension of integration of the sexes amongst patients and staff. Some of the workshops might be good places to start. (Paragraph 7.3.5—see also recommendation 121 below)

9.   There should be a review of the way case conferences are run. This could include consideration of the possibility of relatives in some cases being present for part of the conferences. (Paragraph 7.4.2)

10.   Patients' progress through the 'system' should be reviewed at least annually. (Paragraph 7.4.3)

11.   There should be an improved clinical information system for consultants. (Paragraph 7.4.3)

12.   There should be wide discussion throughout the hospital on the criteria used for determining progress through the 'system'. In the light of these discussions more explicit guidelines should be promulgated. (Paragraph 7.4.4)

Security

13.   When proposals for improvements in patients' quality of life or treatment regimes are being considered, a careful and realistic assessment of the

137

security risks involved should always be made. It should be accepted by all concerned that a certain amount of security risk may have to be tolerated for the sake of the treatment or other benefits which can be gained in return. (Paragraph 8.4)

14.   All staff should carry their security keys upon the leather belt and thong issued for this purpose. (Paragraph 8.5.2)

15.   The practice of leaving security doors open to be locked by members of staff 'following on' should be discontinued. (Paragraph 8.5.2)

16   Security keys should not be taken outside the secure area. (Paragraph 8.5.2)

17.   The deficiencies noted in the control room should be rectified. (Paragraph 8.5.3)

18.   Adequate training should be provided for controllers, watchkeepers and operators working in the control room. (Paragraph 8.5.3)

19.   Security, fire precautions and health and safety at work should be treated as separate parts of the curriculum in the School of Nursing. (Paragraph 8.5.4)

20.   Regular one-day refresher training courses in security should be held for all staff. (Paragraph 8.5.4)

21.   An immediate study should be put in hand of possible ways of introducing a less rigorous security regime in some villa wards. (Paragraph 8.6.4)

Selection admission and assessment
22.   Referring doctors should be actively encouraged to seek the views of Rampton consultants on potential admissions before making formal application to DHSS. (Paragraph 9.1.4)

23.   DHSS should ensure that referring agencies are informed of the way in which the statutory criteria for admission to special hospitals are applied. (Paragraph 9.1.6)

24.   DHSS should carefully monitor continuing trends both in total referrals and in acceptances for special hospital places. (Paragraph 9.1.6)

25.   DHSS should clearly indicate to those concerned that applications for special hospital care for severely mentally handicapped patients will not normally be accepted. (Paragraph 9.1.7)

26.   The possibility should be examined of providing alternative facilities for the physically ill patients at present accommodated in the female admission ward. (Paragraph 9.2.1)

27.   There would be strong advantages in all patients on the admission wards being under the care of one consultant or at least one consultant being specifically nominated as having particular responsibility for ward policies. (Paragraph 9.2.2)

28.   Patients should not have to spend longer than is absolutely necessary waiting for assessment or for their planning case conference. (Paragraph 9.2.3)

29.   The possibility should be investigated of introducing more flexibility into the assessment system. (Paragraph 9.3.2)

30.   Staff should be trained to cover for the Assessment Unit staff during periods of sickness and leave. (Paragraph 9.3.4)

31.   The Assessment Unit should be used as a training experience for newly appointed occupations staff and included in induction courses. (Paragraph 9.3.4)

The organisation of the patient's day
32.   Detailed proposals for changes in the nurses' shift system should be invited from the Rampton staff to enable necessary improvements to be made to the patient's daily timetable. (Paragraph 10.8)

The male block wards
33.   There is scope for further improvements in decoration in the central high security area of the hospital. (Paragraphs 11.11, 12.2)

34.   More could be done to improve the physical environment of the male blockwards, for example by using pictures, posters and potted plants. (Paragraph 11.1.2)

35.   There is an urgent need to improve facilities for private interviews on the block wards. (Paragraphs 11.1.3, 12.2)

36.   There should be a minimum standard of physical amenity in the male block wards, which should reflect current perceptions of what is reasonable. (Paragraph 11.1.4)

37.   There is no justification for the universal practice in the male block wards whereby no patients are allowed to have furniture (other than a bed), pictures or personal possessions in their bedrooms. (Paragraph 11.1.4)

38.   It is not right to refuse to allow all male patients on the block wards the use of transister radios in bed. (Paragraph 11.1.4)

39.   More importance should be attached to male block ward patients having personal possessions more readily accessible to them. The provision of lockers should be re-examined. (Paragraph 11.2.2—see also recommendations 37 above and 160 below)

40.   The arrangements for the provision of razor blades for patients on the male block wards should be re-examined. (Paragraph 11.2.2)

41.   The practice on some male block wards of giving ward cleaning priority over shaving should be re-examined. (Paragraph 11.2.2)

42.   The arrangements on the male block wards for patients changing from day to night clothes and vice versa should be re-examined. (Paragraph 11.2.2)

43.   The way in which bread and tea are served at meal times on the male block wards should be re-examined. (Paragraph 11.2.2)

44.   We question whether patients on the male block wards should have to wear ties at all times. (Paragraph 11.2.3)

45.   We question whether patients on the male block wards should be discouraged from talking at meal times. (Paragraph 11.2.3)

46.   We question whether patients on the male block wards should have to ask permission of a nurse before being allowed to re-enter the dayroom after lighting a cigarette. (Paragraph 11.2.3)

The female block wards

47.   The patients on Victoria Ward should be separated into family size groups with a true staff ratio of at least 1 : 1 throughout the working day. (Paragraph 12.7)

48.   Nursing staff changes on Victoria Ward should be kept to a minimum. (Paragraph 12.7)

49.   All the regular staff on Victoria Ward should be given the opportunity to attend courses and seminars on behaviour on modification techniques. (Paragraph 12.7)

50.   At the earliest opportunity an individual reassessment should be made of each patient on Victoria Ward, in consultation with a clinical psychologist, and an individual programme agreed with each patient's progress being carefully and regularly monitored. (Paragraph 12.7)

Handling disturbed and violent behaviour

51.   After every incident of seclusion, the medical and nursing staff concerned should discuss the events with a view to finding alternative ways of controlling or preventing aggressive behaviour in future. (Paragraph 13.2.8)

52.   There should rarely be any need for an injection when a patient is secluded voluntarily. (Paragraph 13.2.9)

53.   The rules on seclusion should provide for early visits by doctors to secluded patients. (Paragraph 13.2.9)

54. The system of recording seclusion should be reviewed. (Paragraph 13.2.9)

55. The standard of amenity and the degree of flexibility in treatment programmes on the special care units should be as high as possible consistent with the safety of patients and staff. (Paragraph 13.3.5)

The villas

56. Ways should be found of remedying the shortage of private interview rooms on the villas. (Paragraph 14.3.2)

57. A similar facility to the self-contained flatlet on Linden Ward should if possible be provided on the two male pre-discharge villas. (Paragraph 14.3.5)

58. A reduction in patient numbers on Hollies Ward to 20–25 patients would help to allow more individual care and attention. (Paragraph 14.5.2)

59. We hope that at least one more modern villa unit can be provided as soon as possible. (Paragraph 14.6)

Discharges and transfer

60. More thought should be given to programmes designed to prepare patients for departure from Rampton. A more flexible and less uniform security regime should be developed (see recommendation 21 above); the decision which has been taken to set up a patients' workshop outside the security fence should be implemented forthwith (see recommendation 120 below); the rehabilitative function of the patients' shop should be reviewed (see recommendation 163 below). (Paragraph 15.4)

61. The experimental pre-discharge group home training unit temporarily housed in the old Moss Rose school should be extended and continued. (Paragraph 15.4)

62. Outside shopping trips for pre-discharge patients should be encouraged and extended. (Paragraph 15.4)

63. Urgent steps should be taken by the Home Office to speed up their decisions on whether to accept the recommendations of MHRTs to transfer or discharge patients subject to a restriction order. (Paragraphs 5.13.2, 15.5.1)

64. There should be a case-by-case clinical review at Rampton of each of the patients whom data obtained by the Team using the Wessex mental handicap register form suggested might be suitable for discharge or transfer but who do not appear on the official waiting list. (Paragraph 15.5.4)

65. The Eastdale Unit at Balderton Hospital should be retained, and provision should be made for it to take more patients from Rampton. (Paragraph 15.6.3)

66. The possibility of providing a unit like Eastdale for female patients should be explored. (Paragraph 15.6.3)

67. We commend the proposals in Mrs Susanne Dell's report on the transfer of special hospital patients to NHS hospitals. (Paragraph 15.6.7)

68. A joint effort should be made urgently by Rampton and the NHS, with the help of DHSS, to find places for the mentally handicapped patients at Rampton who have been on the waiting list for transfer for more than two years. (Paragraph 15.6.7)

69. DHSS should extend the present arrangements whereby it can make extra-statutory payments to maintain for six months a limited number of ex-special hospital patients in local authority hostels. (Paragraph 15.7)

70. The arrangements described in the previous recommendation might be extended to hostels run by voluntary organisations. (Paragraph 15.7)

The medical staff

71. Rampton should be able to offer better clinical facilities to doctors, particularly in the field of clinical psychology (see recommendation 136 below). (Paragraph 16.2.4)

72. An appropriate fee should be negotiated for RMOs' reports to, and appearances before, MHRTs. (Paragraph 16.2.4)

73. The movement of consultants between the special hospitals should be encouraged, with appropriate upset and removal expenses being paid. (Paragraph 16.2.5)

74. All possibilities for broadening Rampton consultants' experience and training should be throughly explored, including possibly proleptic appointments, sabbaticals, study leave and joint appointments with other NHS hospitals and academic centres. (Paragraph 16.2.5)

75. When consultants are being appointed at Rampton, it should be borne in mind that the medical work at the hospital is by no means exclusively appropriate to specialists in forensic psychiatry. (Paragraph 16.2.7)

76. There should be further discussion towards rationalisation of the role and functions of medical assistants at Rampton. (Paragraph 16.3.2)

77. There should be an increased psychotherapy contribution towards medical work at Rampton. (Paragraph 16.4)

78. There should be discussions between Rampton, local universities and the JCHPT with a view to establishing a part-time senior registrar post at Rampton. (Paragraph 16.6.1)

79. A post of full-time Medical Director should be established at Rampton. (Paragraph 16.7.6)

80. The remuneration offered to the Medical Director should be such as to attract suitable candidates. (Paragraph 16.7.8)

81. A full Medical Advisory Committee, comprising all hospital medical staff, should be reconstituted and should elect its own chairman. (Paragraph 16.7.9)

Other medical, clerical and diagnostic services

82. Urgent steps should be taken to provide an EEG technician. (Paragraph 17.1.2)

83. We commend the establishment of a limited ward pharmacy service, and hope the additional clerical assistance required will be made available. (Paragraph 17.2.2)

84. Drug trolleys should be standard equipment on all wards. (Paragraph 17.2.3)

85. The dental surgery should be re-equipped with modern low-seated functional equipment. (Paragraph 17.3.5)

86. Steps should be taken to eliminate the noise in the dental surgery from compressor and aspirator motors by locating them outside. (Paragraph 17.3.5)

87. There is a need to improve the facilities for radiographic dental examination. (Paragraph 17.3.5)

88. A procedure for the care of dental emergencies should be agreed with medical staff. (Paragraph 17.3.6)

89. An in-service training programme should be established to enable nursing staff on the wards to operate a personal oral hygiene programme for patients. (Paragraph 17.3.7)

90. A dental hygienist should be appointed for two sessions per week. (Paragraph 17.3.7)

91. The catering staff should be made fully aware of the importance of a proper diet in preventing dental disease. (Paragraph 17.3.7)

92. Ways should be found of attracting interest in the vacant speech therapy post. (Paragraph 17.4)

The nursing staff

93. There should be a complete review of the nursing management structure at Rampton. (Paragraph 18.4.2)

94.   Meanwhile the executive authority of the CNO should be examined and re-stated. Management information should be available to him as of right, both as a functional manager and as a member of the HMT. (Paragraph 18.4.2)

95.   A programme of visits and attachments should be arranged for SNOs and NOs. (Paragraph 18.4.3)

96.   More junior nursing staff should be given every opportunity of broadening their experience and being exposed to situations which challenge and develop their existing perceptions of their role. (Paragraph 18.4.4)

97.   There is a case for encouraging distinguished representatives of the health professions and also research workers to come to work at Rampton for periods of time. (Paragraph 5.9.2)

98.   The size of the relief 'pool' of nurses, and the way in which learners and relatively inexperienced nursing assistants are used on relief duties, should be re-examined. (Paragraph 18.4.5)

99.   The style of uniform worn by male nurses should be changed. (Paragraph 18.4.6)

100.   The national agreement on promotion of nurses in special hospitals should be renegotiated forthwith on the lines suggested by Mr Elliott in 1973. (Paragraph 18.4.8)

The School of Nursing

101.   It is essential that the School of Nursing at Rampton should continue. (Paragraphs 5.10 and 19.8)

102.   It might be possible in the longer-term for Rampton to offer basic nurse training for a joint qualification in mental handicap and mental illness. (Paragraph 19.8)

103.   Rampton might also provide the Joint Board for Clinical Nursing Studies' short post-qualification course on the principles of psychiatric nursing within secure environments. (Paragraph 19.8)

104.   Some expansion of the charge nurse complement may be necessary to meet the additional training and service demands implied by the previous two recommendations. (Paragraph 19.9)

105.   The PNO (Education), whilst continuing to report to the CNO, should be operationally independent of him and have complete delegated responsibility for the day-to-day running of the School of Nursing. (Paragraph 19.11)

106.   The control of the selection of students and pupils should be the

responsibility of the PNO, although a representative of the service side of the hospital should always be involved in the selection process. (Paragraph 19.11)

107.　Allocation of learners for training and secondment should be under the control of School of Nursing staff. (Paragraph 19.11)

108.　Discussions should be held to explore the possibility of identifying 'training wards'. (Paragraph 19.11)

109.　Learners should have the opportunity to attend case conferences and case reviews, and the training value of these should be recognised. (Paragraph 19.11)

110.　The hours actually spent by learners on night duty and placements outside the ward should be recorded cumulatively. (Paragraph 19.11)

111.　The amount of overtime to be worked by learners should be agreed and should not be exceeded. (Paragraph 19.11)

In-service training
112.　There should be a radical review of the education and training needs of all staff at Rampton. (Paragraph 20.3)

113.　Substantially more resources must be provided for in-service training at Rampton, perhaps by increasing the staff complement of the School of Nursing but principally by ensuring that the staffing of the hospital adequately reflects an increased training commitment. (Paragraph 20.4)

114.　There should be a substantial increase in the number of nurses seconded for RMN or SRN training. (Paragraph 20.5)

115.　There is a case for organising in-service training at Rampton on a unified basis and appointing a training officer with responsibility for developing and facilitating in-service training for all disciplines in the hospital. (Paragraph 20.6)

Patients' Activity Group
116.　The provision of a hospital radio station should be considered. (Paragraph 21.7)

The resocialisation departments
117.　Every opportunity should be taken of increasing mutual understanding and co-operation between the individual resocialisation departments and between them and the rest of the hospital. Joint in-service training would make an important contribution to this, as would our proposals for a resocialisation team. (See recommendation 169 below.) (Paragraph 22.6)

The Occupations Department
118.　More intensive and challenging occupational activities should be provided for the more able female patients. (Paragraphs 23.4.2)

119.   For both male and female pre-discharge patients there should be a wider range of occupation activities available in low security conditions. The options available should so far as possible be orientated towards preparing patients for the sort of work they might reasonably expect to take up on discharge. (Paragraph 23.4.3)

120.   The decision which has been taken to set up a workshop in a building outside the outer security fence should be implemented.

121.   Integration of the sexes might be tried in some of the workshops, perhaps first on the (female) verandah workrooms and in the (male) pottery workshops. (Paragraph 23.4.3)

122.   Closer links must be established between doctors, nurses and the occupations department. (Paragraph 23.4.4)

123.   DHSS should as a matter of urgency take steps to provide a career structure and realistic pay scales for occupations assistants. (Paragraph 23.5.1)

The Education Department

124.   The problem of lack of punctuality by patients attending classes in the education department should be given urgent attention. (Paragraph 24.3.2)

125.   As a first step towards expanding the educational facilities at Rampton, a special survey of the patient population should be put in hand to estimate how many might benefit from various given levels of additional provision. (Paragraph 24.4.1)

126.   The further education programme should be widened and developed. (Paragraph 24.4.2)

127.   The opportunities for vocational training should be extended. (Paragraph 24.4.3)

128.   Day-time courses could be further developed with courses for example in social and environmental studies, language, literature and art and craft. (Paragraph 24.4.4)

129.   There may be scope for developing integrated social skills and sex education courses for a wider range of patients in conjunction with the clinical psychology department. (Paragraph 24.4.5)

130.   A thorough re-appraisal should be undertaken of the need for group and individual teaching on wards. (Paragraph 24.4.6)

131.   Specialist assessment and guidance for deaf patients, including the services of an audiologist, should be available on a regular basis to the education department. (Paragraph 24.4.7)

132.   Patients should be given better guidance on the education options open to them. (Paragraph 24.4.8)

133.   Teachers should take every opportunity to visit the wards to discuss patients' needs and progress with the nurses, and vice versa. (Paragraph 24.4.9)

134.   Integrated programmes for patients, devised jointly by the occupations and education staff, should be introduced. (Paragraph 24.4.9)

135.   Teachers at Rampton should make and maintain contact with the Home Office Prisons Education Service. (Paragraph 24.4.10)

The Clinical Psychology Department
136.   Clinical psychologists are absolutely vital to the future of Rampton, and this must be recognised by the management of the hospital and by all the staff. (Paragraph 25.5.) Every effort should be made to recruit an adequate number of psychologists (Paragraph 5.5)

137.   Consideration should be given to joint appointments of clinical psychologists with universities or to securing honorary university status for Rampton staff. (Paragraph 25.6)

138.   The establishment of the clinical psychology department should consist of a Top Grade Clinical Psychologist, two Principal Psychologists, a senior clinical psychologist, two basic grade and two probationer psychologists. One of the two basic grade psychologists should be a specialist in work with the mentally handicapped. (Paragraph 25.7)

139.   A male and a female staff nurse should be attached to the department. (Paragraph 25.7)

140.   A technician should be appointed as soon as possible to the department. (Paragraph 25.7)

141.   Adequate secretarial and clerical help should be available to the department. (Paragraph 25.7)

The Social Work Department
142.   We hope that social workers will be able to resume their previous involvement in group discussions, and that some of them will be given the opportunity of further training in this field. (Paragraph 26.3)

143.   The proposal under which a Rampton social worker was, as an experiment, to be placed part-time in a local authority area would be worth reviving. (Paragraph 26.4.2)

144.   There should be a review of the department's staffing levels in one year's time. (Paragraph 26.5.3)

145.   The additional social worker post that has been agreed in principle should be advertised forthwith and raised to the level of second deputy. (Paragraph 26.5.3)

146.   Opportunities for social workers to attend full-time training and short courses needs to be maintained and expanded. (Paragraph 26.5.4)

147.   There should be provision for the regular exchanges of ideas and information with social work staff at the other special hospitals. (Paragraph 26.5.4)

148.   Steps should be taken to relieve social workers of inappropriate routine duties. (Paragraph 26.5.5)

The Administrator and his Department

149.   It should be made possible for there to be interchanges of administrative staff between Rampton and the NHS, and for NHS staff to be seconded to Rampton. (Paragraph 27.1.4)

150.   Professional meetings and training courses in the NHS should be opened up to Rampton administrative staff. (Paragraph 27.1.4)

151.   A decision should be made soon for the phased improvement or replacement of unsatisfactory staff houses. (Paragraph 27.2.2)

152.   DHSS should review the requirements on Rampton and the other special hospitals to keep statistical information. (Paragraph 27.2.3)

153.   The Special Hospitals Research Unit should have as part of its remit the presentation of information about the changing operational performance of the special hospitals. (Paragraph 27.2.3)

154.   Every encouragement should be given to the development of a joint personnel department at Rampton. (Paragraph 27.2.5)

155.   Some form of emergency treatment service should be provided for staff injured on duty. (Paragraph 27.2.5)

156.   There should be a proper occupational health service at Rampton. (Paragraph 27.2.5)

157.   Advice and training on public relations should be made available to the Administrator. (Paragraph 27.2.6)

158.   The standards of service achieved by the institutional services should be known to the Administrator by personal inspection and not simply by report. One of his assistants should also, however, have specifically delegated to him the task of overseeing the work of the institutional services. (Paragraph 27.2.7)

Institutional services

159.   It might be of value to operate the clothing store at Rampton in the style of an ordinary shop. (Paragraph 28.6.1)

160.   All items of hospital issue clothing should be allocated to patients on a personal basis. (Paragraph 28.6.2)

161.   Local management should arrange a regular meeting between porters and car park attendants and a designated member of the administrative staff. (Paragraph 28.7)

162.   New and much larger accommodation should be provided for the patients' shop. (Paragraph 28.8.2)

163.   The hospital should institute a general review of its policy on the patients' shop. There is a case for allowing patients before discharge and transfer to practise using money again. (Paragraph 28.8.3)

164.   We see no reason why pre-discharge patients should not make use of the post office and general store provided for staff in the hospital grounds. (Paragraph 28.8.3)

Management, Finance and Planning

165.   Local responsibility for the day-to-day running of Rampton as a whole should be vested primarily in a Hospital Management Team (HMT), consisting of the Medical Director, the Chief Nursing Officer and the Administrator. (Paragraph 29.4.1)

166.   The Medical Director should be appointed *ex officio* Chairman of the HMT for the first three years of his appointment. After that, the Chairman would be elected by the HMT. (Paragraph 29.4.2)

167.   There should be a Heads of Department Committee (HDC) with responsibilities for the planning of policy and resource allocation. The present Policy Committee should be abolished. (Paragraph 29.4.3)

168.   Attendance at meetings of clinical team meetings should be reduced to more manageable proportions. Teams' main business should be to co-ordinate services for the care of patients. Their involvement in the general management of the hospital should be limited. (Paragraph 29.4.4)

169.   There should be a resocialisation team, whose main function would be to plan the services offered by resocialisation departments to the clinical teams. (Paragraph 29.4.5)

170.   There should be a joint committee of management and representatives of the staff. (Paragraph 29.4.6)

171.   There needs to be an effective system of communication within the hospital. The hospital should seek the help of a body like the Industrial Society

149

experienced in instituting effective communication systems. (Paragraph 29.4.7)

172.   Rampton ought to have a proper staff suggestion scheme. (Paragraph 1.6)

173.   A Rampton Review Board should be appointed by the Secretary of State for a period of three years, charged with the specific responsibility of ensuring that the proposals in this report are instituted. (Paragraph 6.3.4.) During the period of office the Board would have formally delegated to it all the powers over and responsibilities towards Rampton which are at present exercised by the Secretary of State, with the exception of certain reserved powers and responsibilities. (Paragraph 29.5.2.) The powers reserved by the Secretary of State would be negotiation of terms and conditions of service for all special hospital staff; control of admissions; existing DHSS and Home Office powers over discharge and transfer of patients; and determination of Rampton's overall manpower limits and revenue allocation. (Paragraph 29.5.3)

174.   The Board would be required to submit periodic reports on its work to the Secretary of State. (Paragraph 29.5.2)

175.   Toward the end of the three-year period, the Secretary of State should review the way the Board has operated and consider whether any of its features should be incorporated on a long-term basis in the management arrangements of Rampton. (Paragraph 6.3.4)

176.   The Board should consist of five or seven members including the Chairman. (Paragraph 6.3.5)

177.   Some way needs to be found, whether by membership of the Board or otherwise, of associating the Review Team with the Review Board. (Paragraph 6.3.5)

178.   The Board would be serviced by the hospital Administrator and his staff. The other members of the HMT would normally attend meetings of the Board: other heads of department would attend as required. (Paragraph 29.5.6)

179.   The Chairman of the Board should have direct access to the Secretary of State. (Paragraph 29.5.6)

180.   Arrangements should be made through which the knowledge and experience of DHSS officials could be made available to the Board, whether by invitation to attend Board meetings or otherwise. (Paragraph 29.5.7)

181.   The Chairman of the Board should be remunerated on the basis of approximately two days' work per week—certainly during the first year after appointment—and members on the basis of half a day per week. (Paragraph 6.3.6)

182.   The particular needs of the special hospitals should be recognised in the PSA's minor capital programme. (Paragraph 24.6.2)

183.   The system of internal budgetary control at Rampton should be extended and improved. (Paragraph 29.6.4)

184.   Under the proposed new management structure, the HMT should be responsible for financial control and the HDC for the allocation of resources and the preparation of the budget (subject to the approval of the Review Board). (Paragraph 29.6.5)

185.   A policy and strategy statement for the hospital as a whole should be developed and agreed. This could then be translated into an operational plan linked with the annual budget and updated annually. (Paragraph 29.7)

Complaints

186.   The procedure for dealing with complaints at Rampton should provide for complaints to be referred for investigation either internally by the hospital, or by the police, whichever is more appropriate in the particular case. The police may remit a matter to the management or management to the police, after initial investigation. (Paragraph 30.4.6)

187.   Internal investigations should be multidisciplinary. (Paragraph 30.4.6)

188.   It should be made clear that the complaints procedure is concerned not only with complaints which allege physical ill-treatment of patients but with all complaints other than the most trivial. (Paragraph 30.4.6)

189.   The Review Board should take over most of the DHSS's current functions with regard to complaints. (Paragraph 30.5)

Patients, their relatives and the outside world

190.   The booklet produced at Rampton in 1972 for issue to all patients soon after admission should be urgently revised and reprinted, and steps should be taken to ensure that it is given to all new patients. (Paragraph 31.2.1)

191.   More information could usefully be included in the booklet 'Information for the Guidance of Relatives and Friends'. (Paragraph 31.3.2)

192.   There could be organised guided tours of the hospital from time to time to which the relatives of recently admitted patients should be specifically invited. (Paragraph 31.3.2)

193.   There should be early reintroduction of villa visiting and its extension to all the female as well as all the male block wards. (Paragraph 31.3.3)

194.   The new transport department should take an active role in organising

151

the transport for patients' visitors as well perhaps as providing more opportunity for outings for patients. (Paragraphs 28.5 and 31.3.4)

195.   Travel concessions for visitors should be extended to travel by private car. (Paragraph 31.3.5)

196.   Action should be taken to provide improved facilities at the hospital for patients' visitors if it is discovered that there is a demand. (Paragraph 31.3.6)

197.   A measure of flexibility should be introduced into the arrangements for censoring patients' mail. (Paragraph 31.4.1)

198.   In appropriate cases patients should be allowed to use the telephone more freely. (Paragraph 31.4.2)

199.   The work of the League of Friends of Rampton should be strongly encouraged and supported. (Paragraph 31.5.1)

200.   Visits to Rampton by organised groups should be encouraged and where possible new groups should be invited. (Paragraph 31.5.2)

201.   Subject to security considerations and the need to protect individual patients' privacy, Rampton should offer the media every possible facility. The Review Board should take the lead in encouraging openness with press and public, for example by promoting Open Days and the like. (Paragraph 31.7.1)

202.   The media themselves should be prepared to report Rampton in a straightforward and balanced way. (Paragraph 31.7.1)

203.   Less emphasis can and should be placed at Rampton on the provisions of the Official Secrets Act. (Paragraph 31.7.2)

204.   Any necessary restrictions on staff's freedom to deliver lectures or publish articles should be clearly defined and staff should have to do no more than seek the approval of their head of department. Heads of department and consultants should be left to use their own discretion about consulting DHSS or the Review Board. (Paragraph 31.7.3)

205.   Staff should be positively encouraged to give factual talks to local and professional organisations and to write about their professional work in journals. (Paragraph 31.7.3)

APPENDIX A

THE REVIEW TEAM'S TERMS OF REFERENCE

To review the organisation, management and functioning of Rampton Special Hospital and to recommend changes where these are considered desirable.

The Review should in particular cover:

1.   The selection and arrangements for the admission of patients and the establishment of continuing links with relatives.

2.   The general care and well-being of patients together with the arrangements for the safety of patients and staff, and for security.

3.   The nature and quality of the programmes for the assessment and treatment of patients and whether they conform to currently accepted professional practice.

4.   The creation and maintenance of as full a life as possible for each patient consistent with his or her condition and the need for security.

5.   The effectiveness of the arrangements for assessing and preparing for the discharge or transfer of patients who no longer need the secure care provided by special hospitals.

6.   The arrangements in the hospital and DHSS for the adequate monitoring of standards at the hospital.

7.   The general organisation and management of the hospital both within and between disciplines and as a whole, including the role of DHSS.

8.   The formulation of a system for making and dealing with complaints in line with best current practice elsewhere.

9.   The arrangements for staffing the hospital, including the recruitment and training of staff, and the efficient use of staff and other resources.

10.   The links of the hospital and patients with the outside world.

It is essential that the review should not in any way cut across the criminal investigations being carried out by the police for the Director of Public Prosecutions on allegations of ill-treatment of individual patients at the hospital. For this purpose, the Team will need to discuss their proposed programme and methods of work in advance with the Director or his representative.

It is not the function of the Review to collect or consider specific allegations of deliberate ill-treatment of patients. If in the course of their work the Team

153

comes across evidence of such ill-treatment, it will be under a duty to transmit this evidence to the police undertaking the criminal investigation, unless it is clear that the evidence has already been brought to the notice of the police.

APPENDIX B

SUMMARY OF COMMENTS MADE IN STAFF SUGGESTIONS FORMS

1. The Rampton System

1.1   In their general comments, staff clearly felt the potential clash between Rampton's custodial and therapeutic aims. Some thought the system was too institutional and inflexible while others thought that the hospital's primary duty was to protect the public from dangerous patients.

1.2   It was claimed by some that the shortage of teachers, doctors, social workers and psychologists had weakened the multi-disciplinary process. Others said that Rampton did not operate a true multi-disciplinary approach; the nursing staff, via the POA, decided how the hospital operated. Nurses took clinical decisions, eg on seclusion, without reference to other staff.

1.3   It was suggested that patients should be reviewed more often. One patient had not had a case conference for seven years. Junior nurses had little chance to have their views taken into account at case conferences.

1.4   Individual wards should be designated for patients with similar problems, eg arson, schizophrenia, etc, and should experiment with different methods. Another suggestion was that there should be separate wards for the mentally ill, staffed by RMN staff and for less dangerous patients. On the other hand, one person suggested that the behaviour of mentally handicapped patients improved noticeably when they were integrated with other patients.

1.5   It was suggested that there should be female staff on some male wards and that domestic staff should also be employed on some male wards.

1.6   Patients who were re-admitted following discharge or transfer had to start the system again at the beginning. Some wondered whether this was necessary.

2. Security

It was felt that greater participation by staff in patient activities would reduce security needs. Another suggestion was that if perimeter security were increased there could be a lessening of internal security and the introduction of parole type movement between certain facilities, eg swimming baths.

3. Selection, Admission and Assessment

3.1   It was suggested that DHSS should consult RMOs on new admissions. Staff referred to difficulties caused when patients were admitted to Rampton direct from prison within days of their expected date of discharge. It was also suggested that Rampton should have a defined regional catchment area.

3.2   The six-month assessment period was too long and the planning case conference should be held earlier.

155

4. The Organisation of the Patient's Day

Several people thought the patient's day could be extended. One thought this could be achieved by getting patients up earlier in the morning.

5. Patients' Quality of Life

There were several suggestions for improving the quality of life for patients, eg more outings for the elderly, interesting a "show business" personality in organising patients' entertainments.

6. Handling Disturbed and Violent Behaviour

It was suggested that when a patient was 'secluded', the duty medical officer should be informed at once so that he could make an immediate visit.

7. Discharge and Transfer

There should be a 'half-way house' for ex-Rampton patients with full control given to Rampton consultants. There should be hostels near the hospital to enable staff/patient relationships to continue for a lengthly period after discharge to provide a buffer for adjustment to the outside world. Nursing staff should be seconded to spend some time with patients transferred to NHS hospitals in order to support the patient and the receiving staff. Closer links should be forged between Rampton and Eastdale nursing staff. Suitable patients should be allowed a short period of leave after say two years.

8. The Medical Staff and Other Clinical and Diagnostic Services

8.1 Several people thought there were not enough qualified psychiatrists in the hospital for individual psychotherapy, etc. One suggested there should be more medical assistants, as they had the bulk of contact with patients. Others suggested that an incentive be awarded to Rampton doctors to attract better quality staff and that there should be provision for long-service medical assistants to be promoted to consultant.

8.2 There were complaints about the lack of a technician to operate EEG equipment.

8.3 A new drug sheet should be introduced so that a better record of drugs and injections given to patients was available.

9. The Nursing Staff

9.1 Action must be taken to lift nursing morale.

9.2 Attitudes amongst Rampton staff were hereditary and were passed on from parents to children. To break this, it was suggested that more staff should be recruited from outside. On the other hand another view was that because of the patients' unique problems, all staff, excluding doctors and clerical staff, should start as students at the hospital.

9.3 There were general complaints about failures of communication. One group of staff said that "senior staff communicated via bits of paper, but there was no way of knowing what their subordinates thought of the contents".

There were specific complaints that information was not passed from one nursing shift to another. It was suggested that there should be meetings between staff nurses on different wards as charge nurses did not always pass on information to their staff nurses.

9.4   There was dissatisfaction with promotion procedures. It was suggested that any staff should be able to apply for a vacancy at the next level of seniority if suitably qualified. There were complaints that there was no promotion structure in the 'special areas'; 'service area' staff had unfair advantages. It was felt that the division of staff into teams hindered the promotion prospects of nursing staff.

9.5   Staff on 'relief duties', particularly the newly-qualified, got demoralised. They should be carried as part of the ward team as in general hospitals. It was alleged that charge nurse postings and transfers were badly managed and that there were inconsistencies between different parts of the hospital.

9.6   It was claimed that there were too many unqualified night staff. People should not be permanently on night duty; some had been on for twenty years.

9.7   A nurses' personnel department should be set up to allow SNOs and NOs to spend more time in clinical areas.

9.8   There should be an occupational health service or staff medical centre; nurses who were ill had at present to make an appointment to see their GP.

9.9   Recreational facilities for staff were poor and transport should be provided to take them to outside towns for entertainments, etc.

9.10   There were various personal complaints about anomalies in the assisted travel scheme and retirement ages for nurses.

9.11   The wearing of uniforms by nurses was queried. It was suggested that if the present prison officer style uniform for male nurses were to continue, nurses should at least wear white coats on wards. On the other hand, others thought that all staff, not just nurses, should be required to wear some sort of uniform or identification.

10.   Nurse Education

10.1   Some staff questioned whether Rampton was the right place for RNMS training because of the lack of therapeutic practice on the wards and because most charge nurses and staff nurses "poured scorn on the training school". Others admitted there was bad liaison between the school and the wards. Practical training varied according to the personalities, ideals, beliefs and time available from the charge nurse concerned.

10.2   Some thought there should be more opportunity for secondment for RMN or SRN training. One group of staff thought that too much time in training was spent away from the hospital and that learners needed more ward experience at Rampton. Several others thought that 18 was too young an age to start training; this should be raised to 20 or 21. In-service training ought to include night staff.

10.3   Charge nurses who acted as assessors or examiners for the school should receive some remuneration; otherwise the work fell on the few who were prepared to do it for nothing.

11.   The Resocialisation Departments

One member of staff commented, "What I think is lacking in the rehabilitation programme is a basic programme of skills to cope with community living". This view was reflected by others.

12.   The Occupations Department

It was felt that there should be better occupational therapy facilities with more trained staff. There should be scope for occupations staff to obtain suitable formal qualification. Patients should spend more time in the department; they only received 30 to 60 per cent of occupations staff's time each week. There were complaints about the conditions of service, low pay and lack of clear career structure for occupations assistants and of new recruits starting at different points on the incremental scale. Further suggestions received were for a central display area to show off goods made in the department and for a standard form or book to be used on wards to record patients' movements to workshops, etc. It was also suggested that medical staff should take more interest in the department.

13.   The Education Department

Some comments indicated poor relationships between the teachers and some nurses, psychologists and doctors.

14.   Psychology

The shortage of psychologists was seen as weakening the multi-disciplinary team process. It was suggested that psychologists should be paid more, that links should be provided with local universities and that proper accommodation and equipment ought to be provided. There was a lack of goal setting agreements between patients and staff on the patients' therapeutic and rehabilitation needs.

15.   Social Work

It was claimed that the shortage of social workers weakened the multi-disciplinary team process. Social workers' case-work skills were rarely used. One comment was "There always seemed to be friction between social workers and nursing staff, instead of working together".

16.   Institutional Services

16.1   It was suggested that single rooms in the block wards should be given better toilet facilities, heating and controlled ventilation although it was recognised that this would be expensive. There were several complaints about difficulties in getting minor repairs done. Some people complained about the waste of food. There was too much convenience food; more use should be made of hospital-grown produce. English breakfasts should be replaced by Continental breakfasts. Several people suggested it was a waste to issue patients with clothes when they had their own. One person suggested a "topping-up" system for laundry. Another thought more hospital drivers and vehicles were needed.

16.2   Resentment was expressed at the fact that though the staff of the patients' shop were untrained; 'A' grade shop staff earned more than staff nurses. There were complaints that the shop premises were inadequate; toilets were needed. It was suggested that patients should be allowed more time in the shop.

16.3   There were complaints that the finance department was too physically remote. It had many female employees and greater contact with them would help patients' rehabilitation. The portering, stores and accommodation departments were also said to be in the wrong place.

16.4   It was suggested that the standard of staff houses on the estate was low; central heating should be provided as for local authority homes. The redecoration programme was said to have fallen behind.

17.   Management

17.1   There were general complaints about poor communications, remoteness and bureaucracy. Closer liaison was needed between staff and DHSS management. Above nursing officer level, management were 'just names'. Staff views on improving amenities were sought but then ignored. There had been a proliferation of committees on the nursing side since the introduction of the Salmon system. One doctor suggested that a Board of Visitors might be a good thing; it would provide support for staff in times of distress.

17.2   It was admitted that medical management was inadequate. One person thought the medical staff needed a 'guiding light'. Another suggested there should be a Medical Staff Committee with all doctors as members and with equal rights for consultants and medical assistants. There were suggestions for a 'supremo', medical or otherwise. "We have no real leader, just many chiefs."

18.   Visitors

It was suggested thet there should be accommodation at the hospital for patients' visitors to stay in. There were suggestions for providing catering facilities for visitors, for example, a teashop outside the hospital entrance. It was felt that the hospital should have its own bus to transport patients' visitors to and from Retford.

19.   Opening up to the Outside World

It was suggested that the media be used to publicise aspects of patient care. More visiting teams should be encouraged to visit the hospital and play the patients at games.

ORGANISATIONS AND INDIVIDUALS FROM OUTSIDE RAMPTON WHO GAVE THEIR VIEWS TO THE REVIEW TEAM (IN WRITING OR ORALLY)

1. Organisations and statutory bodies

Association of Directors of Social Services
British Association of Social Workers
British Medical Association
Department of Health and Social Security
General Nursing Council for England and Wales
Home Office
Mental Health Review Tribunal for the Trent Regional Health Authority Area
MIND (National Association for Mental Health)
National Society for Autistic Children
National Society for Mentally Handicapped Children
Nottinghamshire Law Society
Prison Officers' Association (Central Committee for the State and Special Hospitals)
Prison Officers' Association (Rampton Branch)
PROPAR (Protection of Rights of Patients at Rampton)
Rampton Hospital League of Friends
Royal College of Psychiatrists
Worksop and Retford Community Health Council

2. Individuals

Mr Geoffrey Ball
Professor John Cooper
Dr D H Dick
Mr James Elliott
Mr G W Furber
Mr Tony Lynes
Dr J G Noble and Dr Peter Sykes
Dr G B Simon
Mr A J Sweetland
Mr Peter Thompson
Dr W J Wigfield
Mr John Williams
Mr John Willis

Note: In addition to those listed above, several people wrote to us about individual patients or ex-patients in Rampton. We also had the opportunity of considering a number of letters and other submissions on general matters relating to Rampton which had been initially directed to DHSS and subsequently referred to us by the Department. We were grateful for all this material. We are also grateful to the large number of people who talked to us informally in the course of the visits we made to other institutions in this country and in the Netherlands.

APPENDIX D

THE AIMS OF RAMPTON HOSPITAL
(HOSPITAL POLICY DOCUMENT)

At the inaugrual meeting of the Hospital Commmittee on 15 March 1972 the following statement of Aims was accepted by the Committee and later endorsed by the Department of Health and Social Security, as a general statement of the Hospital's objectives.

(1)   Under the Mental Health Act, Rampton exists solely for the purpose of treating mentally disordered patients under conditions of special security on account of their dangerous, violent or criminal propensities. For both practical and ethical reasons, it is desirable that in cases where these propensities are not in evidence, steps should be taken, with a view to ensuring that the patient is treated elsewhere or discharged.

(2)   While Rampton is not a penal institution, the staff must necessarily act as the agents of Society in depriving individuals of their liberty. However, apart from the custodial function of preventing individuals from engaging in acts which might be harmful to others, the primary purpose of the Hospital's work should be to prepare patients for return to the community as soon as possible.

(3)   The demands imposed on the staff by the need to prepare patients for eventual return to Society are best understood by considering the problems which patients present. Two broad categories of patient are admitted to Rampton:—

(a) Those whose behaviour has shown them to have tendencies towards aggressiveness, destructiveness or sexual deviation which make them a potential danger to Society at large.

(b) Those whose intellectual limitations or mental disorder prevent them functioning adequately in the Community, but who in addition are aggressive, destructive, self-destructive or in some other way anti-social so that they cannot be cared for in an Open Hospital.

It is possible to identify different treatment and management problems associated with these two groups and the second, although numerically the smaller, certainly poses more immediate problems for the staff dealing with them. The distinction between the two, however, breaks down when the long-term problems are considered.

(4)   The basic problem common to the majority of patients is that they are under-socialised, ie, in varying degrees they lack the normal values, goals and restraints which are necessary to avoid conflict with others and to ensure social acceptance. Inadequate socialisation is, therefore, a main cause of a patient's placement in Rampton, and its correction must be the central consideration for all staff dealing with the patient.

(5)   Deficient socialisation arises from a number of causes, which are at present only partially understood. Basically it implies that at some point in

individual development, the learning of socially acceptable patterns of behaviour has been retarded or misdirected. In many cases, low intelligence is a contributor, though rarely the primary cause since most subnormal individuals achieve some degree of socialisation. In a few cases, damage to the central nervous system plays a major part, both in releasing abnormal behaviour and in hindering normal learning. In some, acute or chronic mental illness may result in a disintegration of previously acquired behaviour patterns. In others, extreme variations of normal biological processes underlying personality may retard socialisation. Finally, exposure to inadequate or inefficient environments early in life, may both facilitate the learning of faulty or inappropriate behaviour, and prevent the learning of socially acceptable behaviour. Various combinations of these can be identified in the Rampton population.

(6)   The central task facing the hospital staff is, therefore, that of providing the necessary socialisation procedures which will effect changes in the patient's behaviour to the extent that his anti-social tendencies are eliminated or reduced. Specifically, this means training the patient in these basic skills which will enable him to meet the demands of everyday social situations and stresses without hostility or anxiety, and with some degree of foresight.

(7) Since both the nature and origins of inadequate socialisation vary from patient to patient, it is necessary to consider each patient's needs individually. Some may require individual therapy, some chemo-therapy, others specific social training, others remedial education or workshop training. Most will require some combination of all of these. It is therefore desirable that there be discussion and feed-back about an individual patient's needs and progress among the various staff involved in his treatment. Group activities, whether structured (eg, work, therapy) or unstructured (eg, recreation) should be viewed as a basic feature of social training for all patients.

(8) The ultimate goal of preparing a patient to a level where he can return to and survive in the Community is an ideal one which may, in practice, be difficult to achieve in many cases for several reasons:—
(a) The present state of knowledge in the medical and behavioural sciences does not permit a clear explanation of all socially deviant behaviour so that the most appropriate socialisation procedures cannot always be specified. Even where the origins of the deviant activities are reasonably clear, knowledge of the effective means of changing behaviour is currently limited.
(b) Some patients' deficiencies are so pronounced that it is unlikely that they will ever be able to function outside a sheltered community.
(c) There are some long-stay patients who present a resettlement problem because of institutionalisation or lack of family ties. Such patients may have already reached a limit in the social skills which they are capable of achieving.
(d) Since Rampton is an artificial environment, there are limitations in the extent of social training it can offer. The changes which may be effected in a patient may be insufficient to enable him to cope entirely with a normal environment.

162

(9)   While these difficulties are very real, they should not be viewed as insurmountable, nor should they give rise to the expectation that some patients are inevitably hopeless cases. Current developments in the medical and behavioural sciences have shown that it is possible to change the behaviour of individuals hitherto regarded as among the most hopeless of Society's rejects. There would seem to be scope at Rampton, not merely for applying methods currently being developed elsewhere, but for exploring new methods of correcting socially deviant behaviour. Even with severely retarded or institutionalised patients, it is desirable that every effort be made to socialise them so that they can at least function in an Open Hospital. Chronic behaviour disordered patients should be reviewed periodically and few patients over the age of 50 should require treatment under security conditions. Some of the problems posed by a patient's transition from Rampton to the Community may partly be overcome by a hostel linked directly to Rampton. If this goal is achieved, it is desirable that Rampton staff be involved at this stage of the patients' treatment.

(10)   As a simple guiding criterion for decision-making involving patients activities it may be useful to ask the following question:—

"Can this particular course of action be reasonably expected to help the patient to learn normal patterns of social behaviour?"

Depriving an individual of his liberty is a fairly drastic step and for humanitarian reasons, it is desirable that this should not extend to depriving him of normal amenities or comforts. However, present knowledge suggests that the most effective methods of changing behaviour are those which emphasise positive and consistent rewards for appropriate or desirable behaviour, and which deny the individual rewards for inappropriate behaviour. For this reason, the indiscriminate use of privileges is to be avoided as much as the indiscriminate use of disincentives.

RAMPTON AND THE SPECIAL HOSPITALS: PATIENT STATISTICS

1. Rampton's current patient population

Table 1 analyses Rampton's patient population at 30 June 1980 (a) by legal status under the Mental Health Act (distinguishing unrestricted from restricted patients); (b) by diagnostic category under the Mental Health Act; (c) by sex.

2. Total patient population of the Special Hospitals: changes 1950–1979

As figure 1 shows, overall numbers in the Special Hospitals have been reducing over the last 30 years. Although this decline is subject to cyclical temporary increases, on the evidence available the general trend is still downwards. Rampton has reduced from 1,100 patients in the fifties to 835 in 1979 although the increase in the early seventies in the special hospital population as a whole had the greatest impact on Rampton, whose population rose again almost to its fifties peak. Since then, there has been a steady and marked reduction. Rampton is still regarded by DHSS as having a 1,050 bed complement although the patient population has declined steadily from this number since 1973.

3. Diagnostic mix of patient population of the special hospitals: changes 1974–79

Table 2 shows the marked increase in mentally ill patients and the absolute and relative reduction of mentally handicapped patients in the population of the special hospitals, and Rampton in particular, between 1974 and 1979.

TABLE 2: *Special Hospitals: Patient mix 1974 and 1979*

| Year | Resident Population | | | | | | | |
| | Number of Patients All Categories | | Mentally Ill | | Subnormal and Severely Subnormal | | Psychopathic Disorder | |
	All Hospitals	Rampton	All Hospitals	Rampton	All Hospitals	Rampton	All Hospitals	Rampton
1974	2,306	1,050	40%	23%	32%	50%	27%	27%
1979	1,995	835	49%	33%	24%	41%	27%	26%

4. Applications for special hospital places and acceptances for admission: 1969/70 to 1978/79

Figure 2 shows that during the early seventies applications for special hospital places were running at about 500 a year until 1976/77 when they fell to under 400. They have remained at a similar level since then. This fall in the number of applications seems likely to have been in response to a similar fall three or four years earlier in the number of cases accepted by DHSS for admission: between 350 and 400 cases were being accepted in the early seventies, but by 1974/75 the annual total has fallen to about 200.

Table 3 shows that within this total declining number of acceptances, the

TABLE 1: *Rampton Patients Resident (30.6.80)—by Legal Status, Diagnostic Category and Sex.*

	All categories			Mental Illness			Psychopathic disorder			Subnormality			Severe Subnormality		
	Male	Female	Total	Male	Female	Total	Male	Female	Total	Male	Female	Total	Male	Female	Total
Unrestricted															
Detained under Section 26	108	101	209	52	32	84	4	5	9	18	10	28	34	54	88
Nominal Section 60-61 / 60	68	13	81	31	2	33	15	7	22	20	4	24	2	—	2
Section 72	13	—	13	10	—	10	2	—	2	1	—	1	—	—	—
Sixth Schedule	36	36	72	5	1	6	3	1	4	9	2	11	19	32	51
Total Unrestricted	225	150	375	98	35	133	24	13	37	48	16	64	55	86	141
Restricted															
Under Section 60/65	308	33	341	89	8	97	138	18	156	79	6	85	2	1	3
Section 71(2) 72 & 73	42	2	44	26	1	27	11	1	12	4	—	4	1	—	1
Sixth Schedule	3	—	3	—	—	—	—	—	—	3	—	3	—	—	—
Other compulsory powers	44	7	51	33	—	33	1	4	5	5	2	7	5	1	6
Total Restricted	397	42	439	148	9	157	150	23	173	91	8	99	8	2	10
Total	622	192	814	246	44	290	174	36	210	139	24	163	63	88	151

165

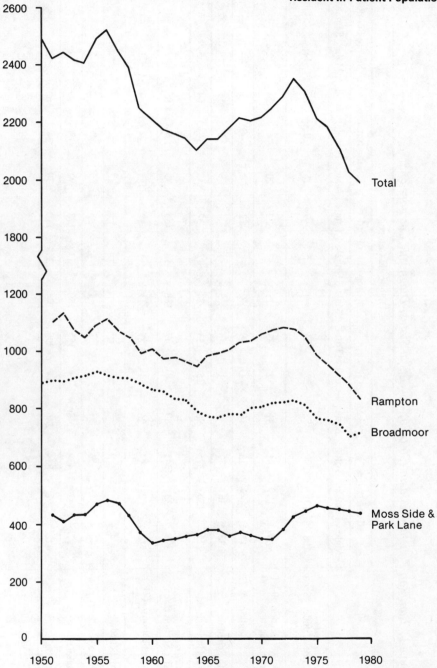

FIGURE 1

**Special Hospitals
Resident In-Patient Population**

Total

Rampton

Broadmoor

Moss Side &
Park Lane

FIGURE 2

Special Hospitals
Applications & Acceptances for Admission

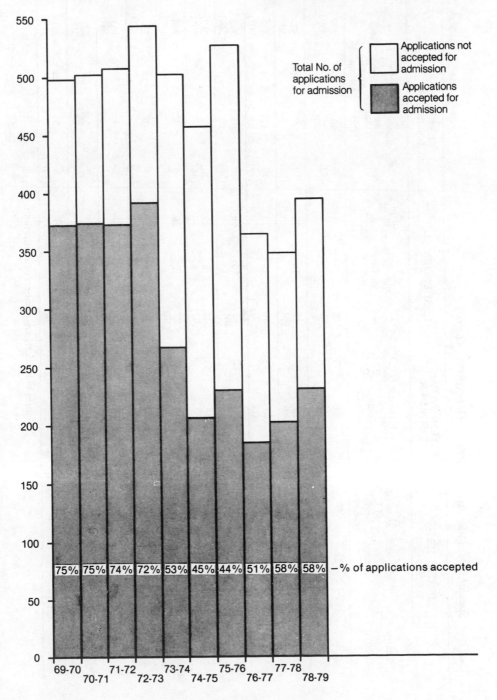

TABLE 3: *Special Hospitals: Acceptances by Diagnostic Category*

Year (1/11 to 31/10)	MENTAL ILLNESS			PSYCHOPATHIC DISORDER			SUBNORMAL			SEVERE SUBNORMAL			TOTAL	
	No.	M.I. as % of Total Accept.	Accept. as % of M.I. Applications	No.	P.D. as % of Total Accept.	Accept. as % of P.D. Applications	No.	Sub. as % of Total Accept.	Accept. as % of Sub. Applications	No.	S.Sub. as % of Total Accept.	Accept. as % of S.Sub. Applications	No.	Accept. as % of all Applications
1969/70	140* (181)	38	77	108 (147)	29	73	87 (123)	23	71	37 (48)	10	77	372 (499)	75
1970/71	155 (205)	42	76	132 (171)	35	77	68 (94)	18	72	19 (32)	5	59	374 (502)	75
1971/72	161 (211)	43	76	102 (143)	27	71	70 (97)	19	72	40 (56)	11	71	373 (507)	74
1972/73	150 (224)	38	67	141 (171)	36	82	63 (91)	16	69	38 (58)	10	66	392 (544)	72
1973/74	121 (213)	45	57	82 (154)	31	53	44 (91)	16	48	20 (44)	8	45	267 (502)	53
1974/75	98 (199)	48	49	75 (128)	36	59	27 (102)	13	26	6 (28)	3	21	206 (457)	45
1975/76	118 (247)	51	48	74 (136)	32	54	32 (111)	14	29	6 (33)	3	18	230 (527)	44
1976/77	105 (192)	57	55	41 (71)	22	58	31 (79)	17	39	8 (22)	4	36	185 (364)	51
1977/78	114 (175)	56	65	55 (83)	27	66	25 (64)	12	39	9 (26)	5	35	203 (348)	58
1978/79	148 (215)	64	69	37 (77)	16	48	38 (74)	17	51	8 (29)	3	28	231 (395)	58

* Figures in brackets are numbers of applications.

168

diagnostic categories have fared differently. Mental illness applications have hovered at about 200 a year and by the end of the decade showed as many acceptances as at the beginning; as a percentage of total annual acceptances mental illness accounts for 60 per cent now compared with 40 per cent formerly. Fewer cases of psychopathic disorder are now offered for treatment in special hospitals and a smaller proportion of them are accepted than formerly. The sharpest decline has been in the two mental handicap categories where applications have reduced by one-third and acceptances by two-thirds.

5. Departures from Rampton: 1970–79

Table 4 gives details of patient departures from Rampton from 1970 to 1979. Figure 3 shows departures from Rampton and Broadmoor per 100 in-patients over the same period and shows that on this basis Rampton's performance is now better than Broadmoor's.

TABLE 4: *Rampton: Patient Departures*

Year	Transfers to NHS Hospitals		Transfers to Eastdale		Discharges		Deaths		All Departures
	No.	% of Departures	No.	% of Departures	No.	% of Departures	No.	% of Departures	No.
1970	63	45			70	51	5	4	138
1971	73	50			63	44	8	6	144
1972	67	51			52	40	12	9	131
1973	66	50			59	44	8	6	133
1974	46	31	22	15	73	49	7	5	148
1975	66	43	39	25	42	27	7	5	154
1976	52	43	31	25	30	25	8	7	121
1977	52	43	20	16	47	38	4	3	123
1978	57	42	23	17	50	37	5	4	135
1979	63	52	11	9	44	36	4	3	122

6. Length of stay of Rampton patients

There are two lengths of stay to be considered; the first is that of the total resident population, and the second the length of stay of those discharged. Table 5 shows the length of stay of the total resident population at Rampton,

TABLE 5: *Rampton: Length of Stay Patient Population*

Year	Length of Stay							
	0–5 Years (% of Pop.)		5–10 Years (% of Pop.)		10–20 Years (% of Pop.)		Over 20 Years (% of Pop.)	
	M	F	M	F	M	F	M	F
1970	56	44	20	22	15	22	9	12
1979	46	30	35	28	15	27	4	15

169

FIGURE 3

Special Hospitals
Departures per 100 In-Patients

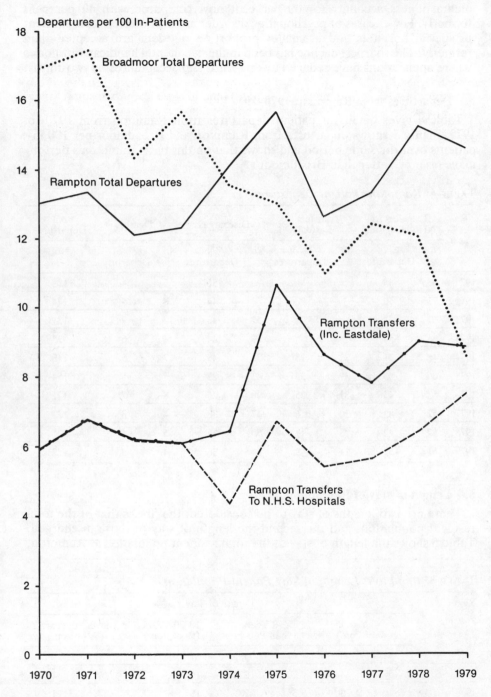

Departures per 100 In-Patients

Broadmoor Total Departures

Rampton Total Departures

Rampton Transfers
(Inc. Eastdale)

Rampton Transfers
To N.H.S. Hospitals

categorised by sex. Only figures for the two years shown are available for comparison; they show that an increasing proportion (for both sexes) have been at Rampton for between five and ten years. The number of very long-stay patients has increased in the case of females but decreased in the case of males.

Table 6 shows the length of stay of patients discharged from Rampton and Broadmoor in 1970 and 1975. Comparision between the two hospitals is difficult because of the different diagnostic mixes involved, but on the whole, Rampton patients (both male and female) tend to have been in hospital longer before discharge than those from Broadmoor. A large part of this difference must be attributed to the generally longer stay of the mentally handicapped and severely mentally handicapped patients at Rampton (approximately 30 per cent or more of whom have stayed for 10 or more years before discharge). Length of stay appears to be increasing but it is not yet resulting in an ageing hospital population which remains predominantly young, as Table 7 shows.

TABLE 6: *Rampton and Broadmoor: Length of stay of patients discharged*

Year	Percentage of Discharges by Length of Stay					
	0–4 Years		5–9 Years		10 or more Years	
	Broadmoor	Rampton	Broadmoor	Rampton	Broadmoor	Rampton
1970	66	46	21	27	13	27
1975	66	46	22	30	12	24

TABLE 7: *Rampton: Age distribution by Sex (31.12.79)*

Age group (years)	Mental illness		Psychopathic Disorder		Subnormal		Severe Subnormal		Total		% in age Group	
	M	F	M	F	M	F	M	F	M	F	M	F
17–19	4	—	3	—	2	—	—	—	9	—	1	—
20–29	52	8	82	17	57	8	18	18	209	51	33	26
30–39	93	27	63	15	35	8	29	32	220	82	35	41
40–49	50	6	22	4	31	4	13	25	116	39	18	19
50–59	26	3	10	—	14	1	9	10	59	14	9	7
60–69	7	1	3	—	1	1	4	12	15	14	3	7
70+	2	—	1	—	—	—	4	—	7	—	1	—
All ages	234	45	184	36	140	22	77	97	635	200		
% of category in Sex Group	37	23	29	18	22	11	12	48				

7. Waiting list for transfer from Rampton

Table 8 analyses the Rampton patients approved for and awaiting transfer on 1 July 1980.

Length of wait for transfer	Total	M.I.	S & SS	P.D.
0–6 months	30 (25%)	10	12	8
7–24 ,,	41 (33%)	14	16	11
24+ ,,	51 (42%)	5	41	5
	122	29 (24%)	69 (56%)	24 (20%)

8. Projection of future trends in the patient population at Rampton

We make four separate projections, based on actual data available for the period 1974–1979 and extending to 1985.

(i) *Projection A* assumes that the average net change per annum for each category of patient over the 1974–1979 period will hold in the future.

(ii) *Projection B* assumes for each patient category for the 1980–1985 period—

(a) the number of admissions per annum equals the average number of admissions per annum during the 1974–1979 period.

(b) the number of discharges per annum per 100 inpatient population equals the average number of discharges per annum per 100 inpatient population during the 1974–1979 period.

(iii) *Projection C* assumes for each patient category for the 1980–1985 period—

(a) the number of admissions in 1980 equals the average number of admissions during the 1974–1979 period and for subsequent years this figure is adjusted annually using the average change per annum in the number of admissions during the 1974–1979 period.

(b) discharges as in Projection B.

(iv) *Projection D* assumes for each patient category for the 1980–1985 period—

(a) admissions as for Projection C except that when in a given year continuation of the process would mean that the number of admissions in the year would either fall below 50% or above 150% of the 1974–1979 average, then the number of admissions in this year and subsequent years are held as appropriate at either the 50% or 150% limit.

(b) discharges as in Projection B.

Figure 4 shows graphically the trend in total patient numbers for each of the four projections.

Table 9 gives detailed data showing the resident inpatient population, both actual and projected, over the period 1974–1985.

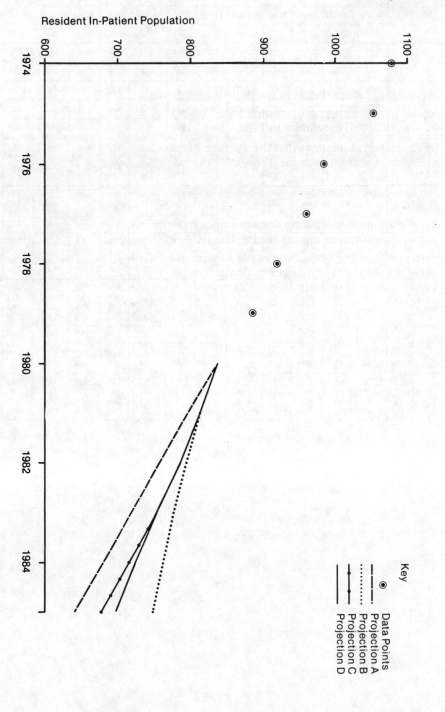

FIGURE 4

Total Resident In-Patient
1985 Projections

TABLE 9: *Rampton: Resident Inpatient Population—Projected to 1985*

YEAR	PRO-JECTION	M.I.			P.D			S. &. S.S.			TOTAL		
		Male	Female	Total	Male	Female	Total	Male	Female	Total	Male	Female	Total
1974		171	54	225	272	38	310	371	172	543	814	264	1,078
1975		185	52	237	255	34	289	364	160	524	804	246	1,050
1976		165	49	214	246	45	291	325	153	478	736	247	983
1977		177	52	229	244	37	281	297	152	449	718	241	959
1978		183	51	234	227	40	267	274	142	416	684	233	917
1979		224	49	273	201	34	235	249	126	375	674	209	883
1980	A	233	48	281	183	34	217	219	118	337	635	200	835
	B	233	48	281	183	34	217	219	118	337	635	200	835
	C	233	48	281	183	34	217	219	118	337	635	200	835
	D	233	48	281	183	34	217	219	118	337	635	200	835
1981	A	244	47	291	169	33	202	195	109	304	608	189	797
	B	233	48	281	179	35	214	205	113	318	617	196	813
	C	233	48	281	179	35	214	205	113	318	617	196	813
	D	233	48	281	179	35	214	205	113	318	617	196	813
1982	A	255	46	301	155	32	187	171	100	271	581	178	759
	B	233	48	281	175	36	211	193	108	301	601	192	793
	C	236	48	284	170	35	205	189	107	296	595	190	785
	D	236	48	284	170	35	205	189	107	296	595	190	785
1983	A	266	45	311	141	31	172	147	91	238	554	167	721
	B	233	48	281	172	36	208	182	104	286	587	188	775
	C	242	47	289	157	34	191	171	101	272	570	182	752
	D	242	47	289	157	34	191	171	101	272	570	182	752
1984	A	277	44	321	127	30	157	123	82	205	527	156	683
	B	233	48	281	169	36	205	173	100	273	575	184	759
	C	250	46	296	141	32	173	152	94	246	543	172	715
	D	250	46	296	144	32	176	156	94	250	550	172	722
1985	A	288	43	331	113	29	142	99	73	172	500	145	645
	B	233	48	281	167	36	203	165	97	262	565	181	746
	C	260	44	304	123	29	152	131	87	218	514	160	674
	D	260	44	304	133	29	162	143	87	230	536	160	696

174

SUMMARY OF THE MAIN RECOMMENDATIONS MADE IN THE ELLIOTT REPORT

1.   Review medical system: clarify duties of consultants and relationship with Medical Superintendent. Consider joint appointments and University links.

2.   Training opportunities in Occupations Department should be exploited more fully (also in kitchens, laundry and domestic work); Occupations Department requires effective leadership.

3.   Rehabilitation departments (psychology, education, occupations and social work) should work as one group.

4.   Need for clearer guidance to nurses and in-service training on reconciliation of therapy and security.

5.   Sisters and charge nurses to be allowed to remain on ward of their choice.

6.   All posts of charge nurse and above to be advertised nationally; short list to be interviewed; introduce appraisal system; all posts above Grade 6 to be subject to open national competition with outside assessor; all service to count in seniority.

7.   Needs of current patients should be compared with and related to basic training.

8.   High priority should be given to expose nurses and others to relevant outside experience through in-service training, study days and visits.

9.   Involvement of all professions, senior and junior, and including trainees in case conferences; review HAS proposals on sabbatical leave and secondments.

10.   Criteria should be established for the length and type of working day which will best aid the resocialisation of patients; trial work schedules which meet these criteria should be developed, tested and jointly evaluated.

11.   Develop a professional executive; discontinue London involvement; weekly meetings; Hospital Committee to appoint own Chairman; miscellaneous recommendations concerning running of Committee; devote agenda occasionally to support services; publish minutes and circulate widely; hold open forum quarterly for informal discussion; Committee to appoint *ad hoc* working parties.

12.   Miscellaneous proposals to enhance the status and role of Rampage (a periodical for Rampton staff and management, now defunct).

13. Gradual steps to an organic style of management with collective professional responsibility at the top but guided by a leader.

14. Local management team to be responsible for managing, DHSS to set objectives, provide resources and monitor results (eg as in relationship with NHS Boards of Governors); replace any member of the team who fails to match up to requirements.

15. Move towards system of budgeting, costing and financial accounting used in NHS. DHSS to make overall allocation of funds but hospital to determine its own priorities; disseminate financial information throughout hospital.

16. Establish a special governing body, accountable through senior civil servants to Secretary of State (as for NHS Board of Governors) but outside the NHS network of health authorities. Board and executive to meet jointly.

17. The so called 'New Deal for Rampton', taking in many of the recommendations listed earlier. Declaration of objectives and policies; a management plan, radical revision of medical system; multi-disciplinary problem solving; a unified resocialisation group; delegation to NOs and charge nurses; re-training with emphasis on therapeutic policies; a fair and open promotion system; major programme of in-service training; experimentation with new work schedules; more devolution of decision making from London to Rampton; a locally based CNO; movement towards a more participative style of management; a greater regard to human relations in personnel policies; the development of the Hospital Committee for consensus decisions; better use of Rampage; better communications between nurses and nurse between disciplines; a top management team committed to continuous improvement.

Printed in England for Her Majesty's Stationery Office by Harrison & Sons (London) Ltd.
07093   Dd 294644   K32   10/80